616-545

000981 X

Pressure Sores – Clinical Practice and Scientific Approach

To my daughter Laetitia

PRESSURE SORES –
Clinical Practice and Scientific Approach

Edited by

Dan L. Bader

Department of Materials
Queen Mary College, University of London

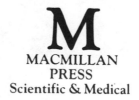

MACMILLAN
PRESS
Scientific & Medical

First published 1990 by
THE MACMILLAN PRESS LTD
Houndmills, Basingstoke, Hampshire RG21 2XS
and London
Companies and representatives
throughout the world

ISBN 0–333–46178–9

A catalogue record for this book is available
from the British Library.

Printed in Hong Kong

Reprinted 1992

Contents

PART II   EXPERIENCES IN VARIOUS CLINICAL DISCIPLINES

Foreword

Robert B. Duthie, CBE, MA, ChM, FRCS

This is a first. This textbook deals with one of the major scourges of mankind, namely the pressure sore.

All aspects – whether in the physical and mental suffering of the involved individual, or in the economics, or in the understanding of the basic phenomena behind the lesion, or in its causation, recognition of presentation and improved treatment modalities – are examined critically and commented upon authoritatively by many experts.

Five per cent of all hospital inpatients, i.e. 30 000 per year, have developed a pressure sore either just before, during or after admission. There are probably even greater numbers in the community.

Twenty-one variables are described which can now be recognised to identify, with a 98 per cent accuracy, those at risk. All health care staff must be taught to distinguish as many of these variables as possible, for example general and systemic conditions of the patient, local conditions of malnutrition, blood supply, abnormal pressures and lack of ability to shift pressures when required. Once these factors have been discerned, steps should be taken to prevent or improve them.

In addition there are several excellent scientific chapters describing known sensors of measurement, techniques of nursing, positioning and splinting.

However, the field of pathophysiology behind the pressure sore is extraordinary complex and diverse and this too has been brought out clearly by several authors.

An excellent chapter for nurses is included which should however also be required reading for all medical students, housemen and indeed consultants. With such a galaxy of authors, including clinicians, epidemiologists and scientists, there must always be some overlap in data and in expression. But this is a multi-disciplinary subject, each discipline with its own language, stretching from a list of homeopathy lotions to the hard science of measuring tissue oxygen levels – for such measurements in absolute terms are required to delineate when cell necrosis occurs at the various anatomical sites.

The fashion of medicine, with all its financial support, rushes on and leaves in its wake the hard core of clinical conditions, e.g. pain, fractures and pressure sores, all producing long-drawn-out and chronic morbidities. This book brings a new look at the field of pressure sores, and highlights

how much more research is required and how badly it is needed. I
recommend it most seriously to all members of the health care team.

Preface

It was with great enthusiasm but not a little trepidation that I embarked on this project. Its major appeal was in its opportunity to develop a structure for a book on pressure sores and select those authors whom I considered most appropriate for the task. This involved lengthy telephone calls with proven experts on both sides of the Atlantic.

There have been several excellent volumes covering the subject area. One such book, *Bed Sore Biomechanics*, published in 1976 by Macmillan, was based on a meeting held at Strathclyde University. Its influence on both the clinical and the scientific understanding of the problem can not be underestimated and is reflected in its many citations in the current volume. My brief permitted me to extend the discussion to include disciplines that have not always been considered important in previous treatises on the subject.

The book has been conveniently divided into four parts involving the clinical, scientific and technological aspects of the problem. The first five chapters consider the general and practical aspects of the subject, with topics ranging from incidence and economics to predictive scales for identifying subjects at risk. These are followed by a series of chapters (6–10) where clinical specialists describe the problems of pressure sores as related to critical groups within the hospital population. Chapters 11–16 discuss the understanding of the normal and pathological processes in the light of basic biological and physical sciences. The last four chapters describe technological solutions to assess subject performance on existing support systems.

In editing this book, I have attempted to avoid unnecessary repetition. However, in some instances certain messages have been retained between chapters. These include the importance of preventive measures and pressure relief for those subjects at risk of developing pressure sores.

The format of the book has been designed to accommodate a wide readership. This will range from individuals involved directly with patient care and clinicians prescribing prophylactic measures to laboratory-based scientists interested in biological control mechanisms. The clinical problem, being ubiquitous in nature, crosses international boundaries and I hope that overseas readers will be able to convert the UK incidences and costs to their own experiences.

My interest in the subject was initiated at postgraduate level under the supervision of Dr Peter Bowker and blossomed during my eight years at the Oxford Orthopaedic Engineering Centre. I am particularly grateful to its director, Mr Derek Harris, for his continued support during this period. Finally I must acknowledge the contributions of Ms Jan Knight and Mr David Grist, who provided the assistance and necessary drive when deadlines had to be kept.

London, April 1989   D.L.B.

The Contributors

D. L. Bader
Department of Materials
Queen Mary College
University of London
London E1 4NS
UK

B. Bailey
Consultant Plastic Surgeon
Stoke Mandeville Hospital
Aylesbury HP21 8AL
UK

J. C. Barbenel
Bioengineering Centre
University of Strathclyde
Glasgow G4 0NW
UK

M. Bliss
Consultant Geriatrician
Hackney Hospital
London E9 6BE
UK

C. Bulstrode
Consultant Orthopaedic Surgeon
Nuffield Orthopaedic Centre
Oxford OX3 7LD
UK

T. G. Burn
Centre for Rehabilitation
  Technology
Helen Hayes Hospital
New York State 10993
USA

K. C. Chung
Rehabilitation Engineering Centre
University of Virginia
Virginia 22903
USA

G. Cochrane
Medical Director
Mary Marlborough Lodge
Nuffield Orthopaedic Centre
Oxford OX3 7LD
UK

M. Clark
Nursing Practice Research Unit
University of Surrey
Guildford GU2 5XH
UK

R. Crow
Nursing Practice Research Unit
University of Surrey
Guildford GU2 5XH
UK

R. B. Duthie, CBE
Nuffield Department of
  Orthopaedic Surgery
University of Oxford
Oxford OX3 7LD
UK

M. Ferguson-Pell
Centre for Rehabilitation
  Technology and
Orthopaedic Engineering and
  Research Centre
Helen Hayes Hospital
New York State 10993
USA

S. L. Garber
Department of Rehabilitation and
 Physical Medicine
Baylor College of Medicine
Texas 77030
USA

I. Gaywood
Department Rheumatology and
 Rehabilitation
Salisbury General Hospital
Salisbury SP2 7SX
UK

H. Gillott
Department of Physiology and
 Biophysics
St Mary's Hospital Medical School
London W2 1PG
UK

A. W. Goode
Consultant Surgeon
London Hospital
London E1 1BB
UK

M. B. Hawken
Department of Neurology
London Hospital
London E1 1BB
UK

P. Hibbs, OBE
Chief Nursing Officer
St Bartholomew's Hospital
London EC1A 7BE
UK

D. E. Hurwitz
Centre for Rehabilitation
 Technology
Helen Hayes Hospital
New York State 10993
USA

C. Khoo
Consultant Plastic Surgeon
Wexham Park Hospital
Slough SL2 4HL
UK

T. A. Krouskop
Departments of Rehabilitation and
 Physical Medicine
Baylor College of Medicine
Rehabilitation Engineering
 Department
The Institute for Rehabilitation and
 Research
Houston
Texas 77030
USA

B. Livesley
Chair of the Care of the Elderly
 (Geriatrics)
University of London
Charing Cross and Westminster
 Medical School
London W6 8RP
UK

T. F. McGovern
Department of Musculoskeletal
 Research
The Cleveland Clinic Foundation
Cleveland
Ohio 44106
USA

R. Masiello
Centre for Rehabilitation
 Technology
Helen Hayes Hospital
New York State 10993
USA

C. Michel
Department of Physiology and
  Biophysics
St Mary's Hospital Medical School
London W2 1PG
UK

P. Noble
Division of Orthopaedic Surgery
Baylor College of Medicine
Houston
Texas 77030
USA

N. Reddy
Biomedical Engineering
  Department
University of Akron
Ohio 44325
USA

S. Reger
Department of Musculoskeletal
  Research
The Cleveland Clinic Foundation
Cleveland
Ohio 44106
USA

J. Robertson
Consultant
Department of Rheumatology and
  Rehabilitation
Salisbury General Hospital
Salisbury SP2 7SX
UK

T. Ryan
Consultant
Department of Dermatology
The Slade Hospital
Oxford OX3 7JH
UK

J. T. Scales, OBE
Department of Research in Plastic
  Surgery
Mount Vernon Hospital
Northwood HA6 2RN
UK

J. Silver
Consultant
Stoke Mandeville Hospital
Aylesbury HP21 8AL
UK

I. D. Swain
Department of Medical Physics
Odstock Hospital
Salisbury SP2 8BJ
UK

Part I
Clinical Aspects of Pressure Sores

1

The Importance of Pressure Sores in Total Health Care

James Robertson, Ian Swain and Ian Gaywood

INTRODUCTION – AN OVERVIEW

At the end of a century which has seen unparalleled advances in science and engineering there remains a number of major health care problems. Two of them are inextricably linked, although at first sight they might seem to be unrelated. They are the problems of pain (Bonica, 1984) and of pressure sores. Pain is a common cause of disablement; pressure sores occur only on disabled persons. Pain and pressure sores are linked by the common factor of movement. Movement, either voluntary or involuntary, inevitably produces postural change. As Sherrington said, 'posture follows movement like a shadow'. The parts of the body in contact with supporting

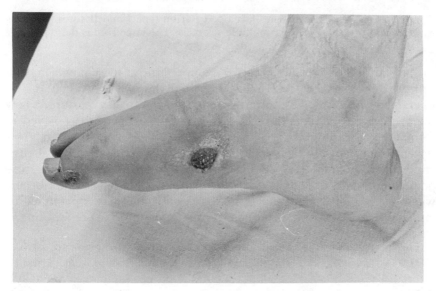

Figure 1.1 Painless pressure sore on foot of young adult with spina bifida caused by a combination of lack of sensation and ill-fitting surgical boots

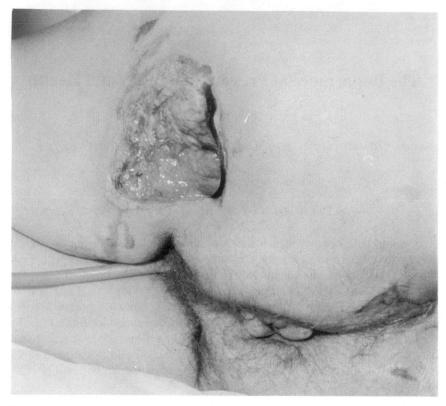

Figure 1.2 A depressed patient developed Barton type I and II sores. She was paraplegic as a result of severe multiple sclerosis. The large sore is the type II or deep sore

surfaces are called pressure points. Pressure borne at these points may be sufficient to produce local ischaemia. In a normal individual this is tolerated only briefly. Discomfort signals the need to alter posture, a new set of pressure points is brought into play and ischaemia is relieved at former load-bearing sites before tissue viability is compromised. This system breaks down if the signal to move is not appreciated, or if, though appreciated, it cannot be acted upon. The former occurs if the pressure point is numb or, of course, in an unconscious patient. The latter occurs when severe pain inhibits movement or the affected part is paralysed or immobilised. Too little pain is as dangerous as too much in predisposing to sores (Figures 1.1 to 1.3).

The major diseases which predispose to pressure sores are stroke (600 000 survivors and 100 000 new cases annually in Great Britain), arterial disease (60 000 leg amputees and 5000 new amputees annually), diabetes, multiple sclerosis (60 000 sufferers and 6000 new patients per annum) and spinal injury. Strong analgesics and sedatives, which may be

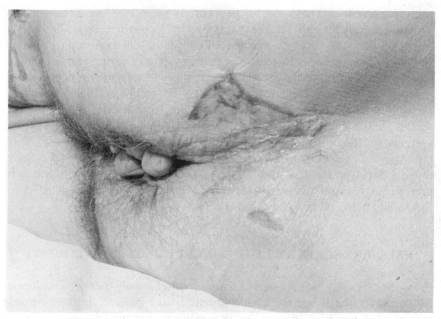

Figure 1.3   This is an enlargement of the smaller sacral sore in Figure 1.2. It is like a friction burn and is a typical type I superficial sore

required in seriously ill, often confused patients, may impair the defence mechanisms described and increase the risk of sores. It has been estimated that 5 per cent of hospital in-patients, around 30 000 patients per annum, have pressure sores. Some are present at admission; others develop during hospitalisation. There may be an equal number of patients with sores in the community. The burden on the National Health Service (NHS) is enormous. The additional cost of a pressure sore complicating a patient's illness has been estimated at £25 000 (Hibbs, 1987a). This estimate suggests a total for 30 000 patients a year of up to a maximum of £750 million. This takes no account of medico-legal costs, which are likely to become an increasingly important factor. In an English court settlement during 1987 an NHS patient was awarded nearly £100 000 for a sore which arose during hospitalisation (Silver, 1987). The increase in legally minded consumerism, accurately reflected in the 300 per cent increase in doctors' defence union fees in the past four years, ensures that this will not be an isolated case. If such a settlement were to be achieved in just 5 per cent of cases of pressure sores in hospital, then the additional bill to the NHS would be £150 million per annum plus the cost of defending these actions. The arithmetic, of course, is approximate, but it serves to demonstrate the magnitude of the problem. The annual cost to the NHS of managing pressure sores may soon reach £1000 million.

Clearly, the most efficient way to manage pressure sores is to prevent their occurrence. They can be prevented, given the resources; if not prevented, they may kill (Baker *et al.*, 1984). The burden is social as well as financial. Pressure sores are markers of care failure. That is not to say that the carers have failed. More often it is the system of caring that is at fault. Carers must be trained in the skills necessary for sore prevention. Money must be spent to allow these skills to be applied. Basic scientists, physiologists and medical physicists have much to offer. The commercial sector should be encouraged to develop and produce patient support systems in the knowledge that the NHS is willing to invest in such equipment. This book reflects three decades of devoted pioneering by nurses, doctors, scientists and industry. Their work has made the study of pressure sores and tissue viability intellectually respectable. This is an expanding field. What follows is but an interim report.

PRESSURE SORES AND THE CONCEPT OF TISSUE VIABILITY

Pressure sores represent localised tissue death. Usually there is a multiplicity of causes, both intrinsic and extrinsic to the patient. Prevention and treatment depend on reversing or neutralising as many of these factors as possible. Only a holistic approach will succeed, since there are as many causes of sores as there are of the death of the whole patient. The concept of tissue viability is central to the planning of a care system for the prevention of sores. In order to understand pressure sores, we need to understand how the fit keep their skin and subcutaneous tissues healthy. Mention has already been made of the feedback mechanism whereby discomfort produces a response of movement in order to redistribute pressure. In investigating the breakdown of this system, we would like to be able to measure three forces, namely, pressure, tension (resulting from the uneven distribution of pressure), and shear (resulting from uneven tensions). Unfortunately, tension and shear cannot be satisfactorily measured clinically. Pressure can be measured, however, and when recorded over time provides a pattern of tissue loading. When interface pressures between anatomical sites and their support surfaces are monitored, force transmissions between the body and the environment are plotted. We are just beginning to measure pressure distribution with time. Such measurements are as fundamental to the problem of pressure sores as are temperature, pulse and respiration charts for patients with fever and blood pressure monitoring for the hypertensive patient. There is of course only one thing that can vary pressure, and that is movement of the body with respect to the environment. Movement is simple to observe but difficult to record. Even more difficult is determining which movements are relevant. The simple answer is that it is only those movements which alter load on the body's pressure points which are important, but this brings us back to

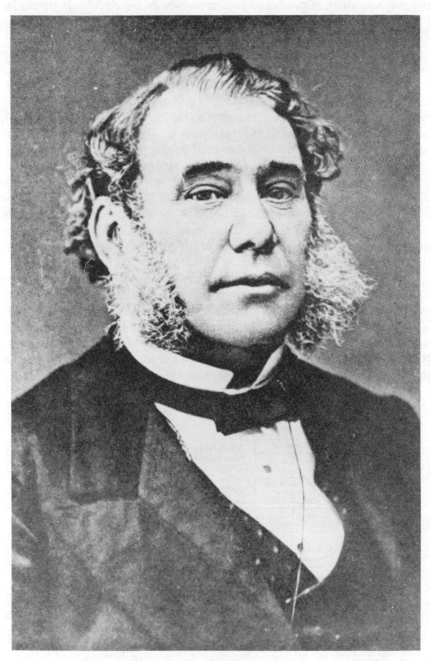

Figure 1.4 John Hilton, 1804–75

the measurement of pressure, so our answer is unhelpful. Of particular importance is movement occurring during sleep, since sleep is metabolically the time for healing and repair.

Movement of the body may be voluntary or involuntary. Distinction between the two kinds of movement must be cautious, since involuntary movement may be rationalised by the mind and so appear voluntary. Discomfort, a very mild form of pain, is probably the driving force behind most involuntary movements, manifest as restlessness. Hilton (Figure 1.4), in his book *Rest and Pain* (1863), said that it is pain which is the primary agent in healing, for it enables the injured person to 'regulate so accurately' and to 'employ so beneficially for his own personal relief and comfort the disturbance or rest to the parts affected'. He was discussing open wounds and mechanical as well as physiological rest. It is important to realise that pain is not always abnormal. Rather it is the absence of this sensation which is both abnormal and dangerous. Ergonomists recognise that discomfort and pain are a normal part of life for many workers, particularly those in sedentary occupations.

So far, several key areas in the study of tissue viability have been mentioned; namely, movement, pressure and associated forces of tension and shear, and pain. Some idea of the complexity of skin tissue viability illustrated in Figure 1.5. It is not intended as a comprehensive representation of the subject. The study of such a complex field and the translation of research data into useful clinical systems for the treatment of sores requires the co-operation of workers from many disciplines.

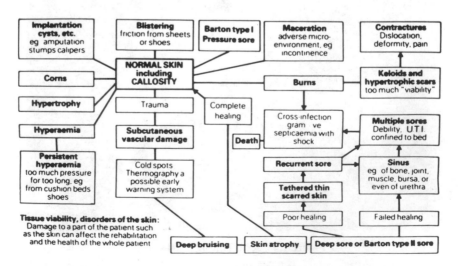

Figure 1.5   Factors involved in the breakdown of tissue viability

TISSUE VIABILITY PARAMETERS

Clinical measurement began in 1700, when Sir John Floyer took pulse and respiratory rates and correlated them with patients' temperatures (Gibbs, 1969). It took another 150 years to understand the significance of fever, the diagnostic evidence provided by charts of temperature, pulse and respiration and their usefulness in monitoring treatment. It does not matter that for a long time measurements were made whose significance was not fully understood. Indeed, if the measurements had not been made the understanding would not have been forthcoming. The pace of science has quickened enormously. Certainly we do not expect to wait a century and a half before achieving an understanding of present-day measurements. Nevertheless, it remains true that without measurement there is no progress.

For some time there was a debate as to whether interface pressures could be measured at all (Robertson *et al.*, 1980). However, today a number of techniques are available (as described in Part IV of this volume), which correlate well with one another. As a result, safe levels of interface pressure have been proposed and certain items used in patient support systems such as bandages, stockings, cushion seats and mattresses have been widely investigated. Pressure relief, below 20–30 mmHg, is the cornerstone of the therapy of pressure sores. Routine measurement of interface pressures is almost entirely confined to wheelchair and seating clinics, where it is used to assess the fit of the cushion and chair to the patient. Ideally, such measurements should be available for the routine assessment of all patient support and handling systems. This would ensure that every health district is aware of the problems of pressure sores and methods for their prevention. Such measurements, made under the direction of medical physicists and bioengineers, should be part of the duty of the district pressure sore teams advocated by the Royal College of Physicians in London in their report (Hoffenburg, 1986).

The impracticality of measuring movement has already been mentioned. Other measures relevant to tissue viability include thermography, transcutaneous oxygen tension, photoplethysmography and laser Doppler studies. These measurement systems should be available from departments of medical physics in every health district. As an example of the clinical application of these techniques, routine use of thermography has been shown to benefit patients admitted to an acute geriatric unit (Davis and Newman, 1981). Every patient was screened for cutaneous hot and cold spots. These indicated areas of damage to the subcutaneous blood supply at pressure points. As a result, pressure point care could be focused on these areas, allowing more efficient prevention of open sores.

PRESSURE SORES AND WOUND HEALING – PATIENT SUPPORT SYSTEMS

Planning the treatment of pressure sores is a holistic exercise. After consideration of the care of the whole patient, including nutrition, discouragement of smoking, continence, treatment of coexistent diseases and attention to psychological well-being, nurse and doctor will have to consider the local care of the wound. This will include a 24-hour review of the physical management of the part of the body affected (Figure 1.6). Nurses have devised 24-hour postural clocks (Figure 1.7), which allow detailed planning of daily life so that at no time is the wound adversely affected by disruptive disturbances.

	Temperature	Humidity	Light	Work	Movement	Tension	Pressure
Dressing	+	+	+	−	−	−	−
Occlusion	+	+	+	−	−	−	−
Support	+	+	+	−	−	−	−
Compression	+	+	+	−	−	−	+
Splint to immobilise	+	+	+	+	+	−	+
Splint in tension	+	+	+	+	+	+	+
Pin traction	−	−	−	+	+	+	−
Rest	−	−	−	+	+	−+	−+
Activity	−	−	−	−	−	−	−
Elevation	−	−	−	+	+	−+	−
Cycled pressure	+	+	+	+	+	−	+
Controlled environment	+	+	−+	+	−+	−	+

Figure 1.6   Physical factors affecting skin with different therapies

Good ergonomics is the basis for the optimal management of disability. For the patient with pressure sores, this means the provision of good support systems. These, besides preventing harm from disruptive tension and pressure, allow easy transfer from one posture and functional situation to another. In designing special support systems it is important to remember that 50 per cent of patients with pressure sores have two or more sores. Many types of support systems are commercially available, their merits being attested to by data varying in quantity and quality. The best data are those derived from controlled trials (O'Reilly *et al.*, 1981; Bliss, 1981). Such trials are difficult to conduct. The multi-centre, collaborative approach used in other disciplines is probably the model to follow.

The treatment and prevention of pressure sores are areas where nursing, physiotherapy and occupational therapy supported by medical engineering services from district medical physics departments and the Disablement Services Authorities (formerly Artificial Limb and Appliance Services) meet. Local social services (housing adaptation and community occupational therapy) and the primary health care team must also be involved. Equipment loan services for wards and community are important (Robert-

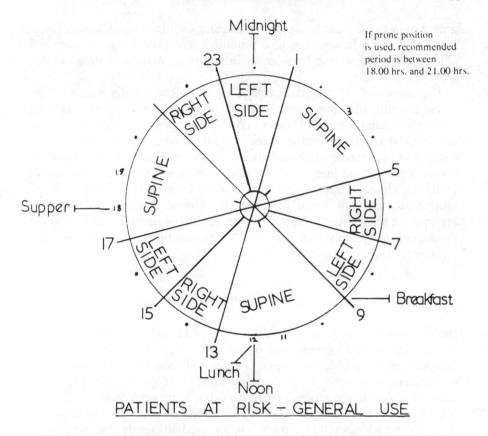

Figure 1.7   24-hour postural clock

son and Haines, 1978). Unfortunately, for such basic services demand outstrips availability; rationing or triage is inevitable. Medico-legally, the provision of less than optimum treatment is difficult to defend. The prevention of sores becomes much more difficult. A relevant, recent legal finding has already been cited.

WOUND CARE

Local care of the wound will start by staging the healing process. Is damage continuing? If it has stabilised, has dead material been removed where appropriate? Debridement may be surgical, enzymatic or by lavage. A clean wound should granulate well. Granulation tissue is the basis of healing, for it fills the wound and draws it together. It provides the medium for growth of new blood vessels and the surface for the growth of new skin across the wound. A shortage of oxygen may promote the formation of granulation tissue but also increases the risk of infection. A wet environment may speed healing but also promotes infection. Surgeons may feel able to close the wound by primary intention or may offer delayed skin grafting.

The science of wound management has advanced rapidly from passive, often harmful, dressings combined with traditional and equally harmful antiseptics (Cameron and Leaper, 1987) to the present range of reactive dressings which absorb moisture and control the wound environment while being non-adherent and thus allowing almost pain-free removal. In the future there will be interactive dressings which will stimulate the wound with trace elements and trophic hormones while protecting it with disinfectants which do not harm cell growth. Wound healing systems may incorporate skin tissue cultures. Further, careful evaluation will lead to the production of systems with improved characteristics of compression, and moisture and thermal control.

MANAGERIAL ASPECTS OF SORES

No mention has yet been made of the role of Health Service managers in the prevention and management of pressure sores. An awareness among managers of the problem of pressure sores and their financial implications is essential. Resources are limited and must be competed for. Managers must also realise that pressure sores often represent failures of care. Clinicians are becoming accustomed to audit, essentially a gathering of data to determine whether money is being used efficiently. Measures such as the rate of presentation of pressure sores in a district, the rate of sore generation while patients are in the care system, the rates of healing and of recurrence may well be used in this way. If managers are to use such data sensibly and draw the right conclusions from them they must have some background knowledge of the problem. Once the problem has been quantified in a district it will be possible to document changes in these parameters. In this way a set of performance indicators can be derived with which to measure progress. Different districts, and therefore different care systems, will be compared. Perhaps we will derive standardised sore rates in the same way in which we now derive standardised mortality rates, paying particular attention to standardisation for age.

THE TISSUE VIABILITY SOCIETY

In any area which brings together professionals from a wide range of backgrounds there is a need for a forum for debate, the exchange of knowledge and the establishment of common goals. The Tissue Viability

Society and its journal, *Care, Science and Practice*, satisfy these needs. The Society is independent of the NHS, allowing views to be expressed with less inhibition. The existence of such a forum will enhance the rate of progress in the field. It also does much to remove the sense of isolation of those working in an apparently unglamorous area.

The scientific problem of pressure sores has been tacked to great effect. Most sores could be prevented if present knowledge was applied. What limits progress? Probably the effectiveness of management, whose prime task must be to achieve adequate resources and be able to demonstrate that these are being used efficiently (Hibbs, 1987b).

REFERENCES

Baker, J. H. E., Silver, J. R. and Tudway, A. J. C. (1984). Late complications of pressure sores. *Care, Science and Practice*, **3**, 56–59

Bliss, M. R. (1981). Clinical research in patient support systems. *Care, Science and Practice*, **1**, 17–36

Bonica, J. J. (1984). In Kruger, L. and Liebeskind, J. C. (eds), *Advances in Pain Research and Therapy*, Vol. 6, Raven Press, New York, pp. 1–22

Cameron, S. and Leaper, D. (1987). Antiseptic toxicity in open wounds. *Care, Science and Practice*, **5**, 19–20

Davis, N. H. and Newman, P. (1981). Skin temperature measurements with regard to pressure sores and their development. *Care, Science and Practice*, **1**, 46–49

Gibbs, D. D. (1969). Sir John Floyer, MD (1649–1734). *British Medical Journal*, **1**, 242–245

Hibbs, P. J. (1987a). Strategies for the elimination of pressure sores. *Care, Science and Practice*, **5**, 15–19

Hibbs, P. J. (1987b). Paper presented to the Tissue Viability Society, Guildford, 28–29 September 1987

Hilton, J. (1863). In Walls, E. W. and Phillip, E. E. (eds), *Hilton's Rest and Pain* (1950), Bell, London, p. 4

Hoffenburg, R. (1986). Physical disability in 1986 and beyond. A committee report. *Journal of the Royal College of Physicians*, **20**(3) 161–193

O'Reilly, M. O., Whyte, J. and Goldstone, L. (1981). Pressure sore survey. *Nursing Times*, Supplement, 30 September, 7–19

Robertson, J. C. and Haines, J. R. (1978). A community/hospital home aids loan scheme (based on a rehabilitation demonstration centre). *Health Trends*, **10**, 15–16

Robertson, J. C., Shah, J., Druett, J. E. and Gisby, J. (1980). An interface pressure sensor for routine clinical use. *Engineering in Medicine*, **9**, 151–155

Silver, J. (1987). Letter. *Care, Science and Practice*, **5**, 30

2

Pathogenesis of Pressure Sores

J. T. Scales

INTRODUCTION

Healthy man is a dynamic person who does not develop decubitus ulcers or bed sores. Throughout a healthy life the body is not motionless for a long enough period, day or night, for forces of sufficient magnitude and duration to act on the tissues in such a manner as to cause tissue damage. Human pressure sores are a manifestation of immobility due to anaesthesia or sedation, disease or injury, resulting in diminished pain sensation and/or diminished musculoskeletal activity.

Decubitus ulcers, bed, distortion or pressure sores, are reported in 3 per cent to 9.4 per cent of hospital patients (Petersen *et al.*, 1971; Jordan *et al.*, 1977). The monetary cost in the United Kingdom was estimated in 1982 at £150 million per annum (Scales *et al.*, 1982). By the year 2025, 25 per cent of the population will be over 65 years of age. Besides causing untold patient suffering and even death, the occurrence of pressure sores often delays the discharge of the patient from hospital, thus reducing the efficiency of the Health Service.

Young and Burns (1982) stated that 'The injured person may be further confronted with the tragedy of a foul, saucer-sized, bone deep sore. His marginal metabolism must deal with the added insult of such things as nitrogen imbalance, hypoproteinemia and sepsis. His psyche is overwhelmed with revulsion. What next?'

The pressure sore is the result of impairment of the vascular and lymphatic systems of the skin and deeper tissues caused by the development of compression, tension and shear forces above a critical value and acting for a critical period of time in the tissues between the skeleton and a surface supporting the body. Many other extrinsic and intrinsic factors associated with the condition and nursing of the patient facilitate the development of this type of tissue injury and are discussed in other chapters.

The prevention of pressure sores requires an appreciation of the structure of the skin and the deeper tissues and their blood supply, and the physical effects in the tissues produced by the structures which may support a patient.

STRUCTURE AND FUNCTION OF HUMAN SKIN

The skin (Figure 2.1) is the largest organ of the body and performs a number of vital functions. It is the waterproof but water-vapour- and gas-permeable covering that protects the body against mechanical damage, excess ultraviolet radiation and infection. Some exposure to ultraviolet radiation is, however, necessary for the synthesis of vitamin D, the major source of which is the skin. The fat, stored in the innermost layer, sweat glands and about 90 per cent of the vascular system are concerned with temperature regulation. It is a major sensory organ, with a variety of sensory nerve endings, which not only protects the body from mechanical and thermal injury but also allow tactile discrimination. It consists of three layers: the epidermis, the dermis and the hypodermis or subcutaneous tissue. There is a considerable variation in the relative thickness of the layers in the different parts of the body. The epidermis is thickest on the sole of the foot and the palm of the hand, the dermis and hypodermis on the back and the hypodermis on the buttock.

Epidermis

The epidermis, which is derived from embryonic ectoderm, is avascular. Its outer layers are dead keratinised cells, chemically inactive, arranged parallel to the surface of the body, derived from the proliferating basal cell layer of the epidermis adjacent to the dermis. For the proper maturation of the water-vapour-permeable epidermis, dehydration of the keratinocytes is essential. The maintenance of the normal bacterial flora of the skin also requires that normal dryness of the skin is maintained and thus materials in contact with the skin must be water vapour permeable. Important extensions of the epidermis that pass into the dermis and the adipose hypodermis are the hair follicles, with their associated arrector pili muscles and apocrine glands, and the sweat or eccrine glands.

Dermis

The dermis, mesenchymal in origin, is a highly vascular tissue, well supplied with sensory receptors to pain, temperature and touch. It contains two types of connective tissue: high-tensile-strength white fibrous collagenous connective tissue and yellow elastin connective tissue, which provides skin with its characteristic recovery following stretching. The mechanical properties of these compounds diminish with age. Between the connective tissue fibres is a mucopolysaccharide ground substance the viscosity of which is variable. The epidermis is stabilised on the dermis by the downward

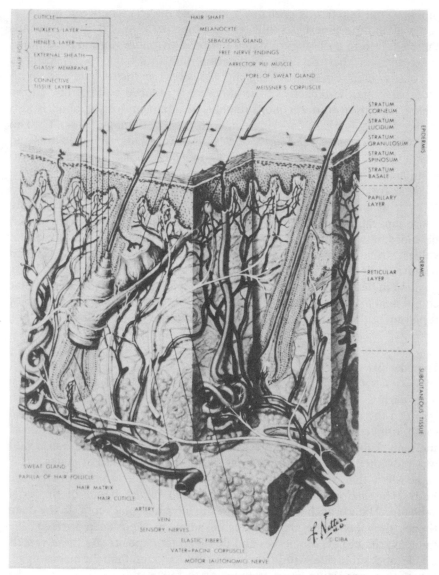

Figure 2.1 Structure of skin (drawing by F. Netter reproduced by kind permission of Ciba Foundation from *Ciba Clinical Symposia 1967*, **19**(2), 38)

projections of the epidermis, rete pegs, which follow the convolutions of the papillary dermis. This arrangement of the dermal–epidermal junction, with the surplus of epidermal cells in the rete pegs, facilitates normal flexion and extension of the skin without separation of the two structures or splitting of the epidermis. While extensions of basal cell cytoplasm have been described which extend into the dermis at the dermo-epidermal junction, the junction is probably a chemical interface between the basal cell wall and the superficial collagen, allowing passage of dermal cells into the epidermis in pathological states and possibly under normal conditions. It would seem that the dermal–epidermal interface behaves physically as an oily viscous bond providing an adhesive for the two layers. With increasing age the tenacity of the adhesive is reduced and thereby allows blister formation to occur more readily. The tenacity of the bond is also reduced with increase in skin temperature in the range 20–40 °C. The interface is not penetrated by blood vessels or lymphatics. Nerve fibres and elastic fibres pass from the dermis to the basal cells and may help to maintain the cohesion of the epidermis and dermis (Jarrett, 1973).

Shear forces can be applied to the epidermis, as in the use of garden tools or when a person slides on a surface. These forces do not normally cause separation of the dermal–epidermal junction unless the friction that develops between the epidermis and the contact surface reaches abnormal values, when the tissue water blister occurs. These values can be reached when a patient is dragged rather than lifted into a comfortable sitting position in bed. The structure of the dermis and epidermis, and the cellular components of the dermis, combat infection and provide the means of repairing both superficial and deep wounds of the skin.

Hypodermis

The dermis and hypodermis are stabilised by the irregular junction between the compact connective tissue of the dermis and the adipose and loose connective tissue of the hypodermis. In 1988 an English translation of the remarkable studies of Professor Michel-Marie Salmon (Salmon, 1936) was published with the title *Arteries of the Skin*. The author states, 'It is established that vessels follow the connective tissue framework of the body. The major arteries are closely related to the bones of the axial skeleton. Their branches at first follow the intramuscular septa. In the deep tissues they penetrate the muscles, usually on their deep surface, the tendons, the bones, the nerves and the deep fat deposits. As these vessels divide and subdivide within the specialised tissues their branches again follow the connective tissue framework to reflect the architecture of the tissue in question, a relationship which can be traced to the microscopical level. The cutaneous perforators exhibit the same pattern. They arise from the source artery or one of its muscular branches and follow inter- or intra-muscular septa towards the surface. They pierce deep fascia, branch and ramify on its surface.' Those vessels which are deep to the hypodermis are essentially parallel to the surface of the skin. Branches find their way between the fat globules to anastomose in the capillary network of the dermal papillae adjacent to the basal cell layer. There is a particularly rich capillary supply to the sweat glands and the base of the hair follicles.

As can be seen from Figure 2.1, the arrangement of the blood supply is particularly suited to the effect of pressure on the skin in that branches from the deeper vascular system become more coiled initially when direct pressure is applied to the skin surface, thus limiting the risk of occlusion. A bony prominence below the vessels running parallel to the surface of the skin may, however, increase the risk of occlusion of the deeper vessels running parallel to the surface of the skin. Further, if excessive shear within the tissues is induced, such as when a patient propped up in bed tends to slide down the bed on a wrinkled sheet covering a waterproof non-water-vapour-permeable plastics mattress cover, traction of the vessels will occur with potential disruption of the dermal–epidermal junction. This situation should never be allowed to arise in hospital, since by the simple expedient of tilting up the foot of the bed by some 10 ° there is a marked reduction in the magnitude of the induced shear forces within the tissues and at the surface of the skin.

The adipose tissue of the hypodermis is a thermal insulator and, like all other tissues, has energy absorbing properties. The skin, in common with all biological tissues, is a viscoelastic structure, i.e. it has a viscous component by virtue of its fluid content and an elastic component due to the fibres of elastin interwoven with the collagen of the dermis. Under sustained load, because of their viscous property, the tissues creep or flow and when the load is removed the tissues take a period of time to return to their original form. The viscoelastic phenomenon is clearly seen when pressure is removed from oedematous tissue. With increasing age the elastin content diminishes and there is a relative increase in the viscous component. Except over bones, such as the sacrum and tibia, the skin is freely movable on a layer of areolar tissue that overlies the deep fascia.

CAUSATION OF PRESSURE OR DISTORTION SORES

It has taken many years of clinical observation and trial of methods of patient care, coupled with laboratory and clinical experiments, to establish the cause of pressure sores. Because of the interrelation of the various observations and findings, the following is written as a continuum.

In 1853 Brown-Sequard (1853) showed that in experimental animals with paraplegia pressure sores could be healed and prevented if the skin was not subject to periods of sustained pressure, thus establishing that pressure sores were not directly related to the neurological damage. Paget (1873) maintained that sustained pressure on the tissues was the primary cause of pressure sores and 'they will, of course, be accelerated by dirt if his urine and faeces are not constantly removed.' Trumble (1930) found that when local pressures of about 78 mmHg (10.4 kPa) were applied to the skin, patients complained of pain and that while these pressures did not cause collapse of large arteries, veins and capillaries were so affected.

Cattell (1936) investigated the effect of hydrostatic pressure on unicellular organisms and found that pressures in excess of 1.3×10^9 mmHg (173 GPa) were required before significant changes in cellular function were observed, indicating that the role of pressure in the formation of pressure sores is to restrict circulating fluid. Pressure sores do not occur in deep-sea diving because the external pressure which develops as the depth of the dive increases is balanced by the increasing pressure of the gases breathed, and hence the tissues become increasingly pressurised, resulting in no pressure differential between the tissues and the applied external pressure.

Munro (1940), in a paper on the care of the back following spinal-cord injuries, stated that 'pressure sores only develop because of secondary destruction of local tissues. The occurrence and extent of the destruction depends on the presence of a bony weight-bearing prominence close beneath the skin, the thickness of the padding tissue between the bone and skin itself, the length of time that constant weight bearing is permitted over the point and the integrity of the protective horny layers of the skin . . . There must be in addition a local anoxia and anaemia.' His experience indicated that the only therapeutic essentials to preventing the development of pressure sores were to move the patient on an exact hourly time schedule, to avoid all forms of external artificial splint or support to the spinal column so long as the patient is bedridden, to prevent sepsis or exhaustion, to keep the patient constantly and completely dry, and the use of a sponge rubber mattress.

Groth (1942) differentiated between two forms of pressure sore of essentially different anatomical origin. Those which developed in the skin he described as the benign form, while those originating in muscle he termed the malignant form. The latter are the result of a process which begins in deep tissue such as muscle and then spreads to the surface after the necrotic tissue deep in the hypodermis becomes infected by blood-borne organisms. Using three groups of rabbits, he studied the effect of constant local pressure on the gluteal muscle of healthy normal, infected and paralysed animals. Constant local pressure above 24 mmHg (3.2 kPa) applied to rabbits of about 2 kg mass led to irreversible degenerative changes and capillary haemorrhages in muscle, followed by necrosis. The skin on which the pressure was directly exerted was not noticeably affected for upward of 90 minutes to 3 hours. In those animals infected with staphylococci or streptococci there was purulent liquefaction of the necrotic tissues. No significant differences were noted in experiments on animals with flaccid paralysis following division of the spinal cord compared with those on healthy animals, although it was noted that atony and vasomotor disturbances associated with the flaccid paralysis enhance the effect of local pressure.

In 1948 Gardner and Anderson, quoting Munro, described an alternating pressure support system consisting of air cells 32 mm in diameter running transversely to the length of the mattress. Alternate air cells were inflated and deflated at intervals of 2 to 3 minutes so that the patient's body was resting on the odd-numbered cells and then on the even-numbered ones. This produced a massaging effect, which was believed to aid cutaneous circulation, the alternate inflation and deflation of the system being achieved by a pump driven by a $\frac{1}{150}$-horsepower (5.0 W) motor. The inflation pressure was approximately 50 mmHg (6.7 kPa). Since that time the alternating-pressure or ripple mattress employing pressures up to 90 mmHg (12 kPa) has been widely used throughout the world, demonstrating that pressure sores can be prevented if the vascular and lymphatic systems in tissues both superficial and deep are not compromised for more than 4 to 5 minutes. More recently, because of criticism of the effectiveness of the large-cell ripple mattress and its ancillary equipment, a two-layer ripple cell system has been described in which every third cell in turn is deflated, each cycle taking 7.5 min (Exton-Smith *et al.*, 1982). The mattress is ventilated by numerous fine holes, through which air passes to help ventilate the skin. The air is dispersed by a washable wool fleece placed on top of the mattress. A plastics drawsheet is not used as this would impair ventilation of the skin. It is claimed that in clinical trials the system is more effective than the large-cell ripple mattress in preventing and reducing the severity of pressure sores and in promoting recovery from existing sores.

Husain (1953) again pointed out that when pressure is evenly distributed over a wide area of the body, damage is far less than when the total pressure has to be sustained by localised areas of the body surface. However, the same localised high pressures sustained for frequent short periods of time will result in less or even no damage. Pressure sores may originate not only in the skin over bony prominences such as the occiput, the sacrum, the trochanter, the inner condyle of the knee, the medial malleolus and the heel, but also in muscle masses such as the glutei and the calf. Guttmann (1953) in his detailed paper on the treatment and rehabilitation of patients with injuries of the spinal cord stated that 'intrinsic and extrinsic factors determining the formation of bed sores can be distinguished. The most important intrinsic factor is the lowering of the tissue resistance to pressure during the stage of spinal shock when, as a result of the acute interruption of the spinal vasomotor pathways, there results a flaccid paralysis of muscle associated with loss of vasomotor control.' With this condition there is a gradual loss of muscle bulk with greater risk of distortion of the vascular and lymphatic systems.

Kosiak (1959), using dogs, found that ischaemic ulcers were produced both by high pressures applied for a short duration and by low pressures applied for a long duration. The time–pressure relationship is converse and follows a parabolic curve. Microscopic pathological changes were noted in tissues subject to 60 mmHg (8 kPa) for one hour. Kosiak stated that because living tissues are so sensitive to ischaemia produced by very low external pressures, temporary relief of this pressure every few minutes is essential.

Hickman *et al.* (1966) reported on studies of deformation and flow in compressed skin. The level and duration of pressures applied to the tissue were typical of everyday life and did not cause any significant tissue damage. Using a creep test which measured the tissue response to constant prolonged pressure, they were able to measure the two components of response: instantaneous elastic compression followed by creep deformation. When the load was removed there was an instantaneous elastic recovery followed by viscoelastic recovery.

Ageing in man causes significant changes in rheological behaviour and response to pressure in that there is a reduction in amount of instantaneous elastic compression and delayed elastic recovery (Bader and Bowker, 1983). Delayed elastic compression and moulding deformation are increased. This agrees with the clinical observations that elasticity of skin is reduced and the ground substance becomes more viscous with advancing years. While the tissues offer more immediate resistance to compression, there is an increased tendency to deform with constant pressure and recovery is delayed after removal of pressure. Oedematous tissue was found to be more deformable than normal tissue and moulding behaviour was more pronounced with loss of elasticity. In obesity, creep tests showed that fatty tissue is more elastic than normal tissue. When compressed it immediately deformed by a greater amount than normal tissue, the deformation being essentially compression and displacement with little viscous flow. The general patterns of rheological behaviour were found to be similar in skin tissues in various parts of the body and in both humans and animals. External pressures well above capillary pressure applied for a few minutes did not compromise blood flow, but when more moderate pressures of 40 mmHg (5.3 kPa) were applied for periods of 30 to 60 minutes blood flow was seriously impaired owing to deformation by creep of the tissues. The studies reported, coupled with those of Daly *et al.* (1976), Vogel (1977), Cochran (1979) and Reddy *et al.* (1981), indicate that in the prevention of ischaemia it is important to prevent the flow of interstitial fluids and the mucopolysaccharide ground substance by limiting deformation or distortion of tissues.

Palmer *et al.* (1968) discussed the effect of pressure and shear generated on body surfaces in relation to the tissue damage. They concluded that, while shear stress alone had no particularly damaging quality, its interaction with other tissue forces could produce damage in the tissues which was different from that induced by direct pressure. They also stated that, after longer periods of exposure to pressure, adding a shear force component appeared to reduce the superficial ulcerating effect of normal pressure at

60 mmHg (8 kPa). This finding contrasts with that of Bennett *et al.* (1979), who found that the combination of pressure with shear was particularly effective in promoting blood flow occlusion. At a shear stress of approximately 75 mmHg (10 kPa) the pressure required to produce arterial occlusion was reduced by a factor of two.

Bader *et al.* (1986), who studied the effect of externally applied skin surface forces on tissue vasculature, found that with a mean force intensity of 1.3 N/mm and a strain of 10 per cent it was possible to achieve virtual obliteration of blood flow to the capillaries. It was pointed out that with a 70 kg patient lying in bed with the trunk inclined at 30 ° to the horizontal and with a sacral contact width of 300 mm, the force intensity at the sacrum is approximately 0.6 N/mm. This value was shown to be sufficient to significantly reduce capillary blood flow. When lying in bed at this angle, the patient tends to slide towards the foot end of the bed. To reduce this tendency and to reduce the force intensity at the sacrum, the foot end of the bed should be raised 5–10 °.

Husain (1953) found that a pressure of 100 mmHg (13.3 kPa) applied to skin for 2 hours produced signs of pressure damage in the tissues. He also noted that with oedema poor lymphatic function with clogging of lymphatics was associated with sore formation. Krouskop *et al.* (1978) suggested that the application of mechanical loads impairs the function of the contractile lymphatic system and that the impairment of the lymphatic function combined with change in the microvascular system of the skin causes accumulation of metabolic waste products in the tissues. They pointed out that lymphatic occlusion resulting in oedema occurs with subcutaneous pressures in excess of 60 mmHg (8 kPa). This is discussed further in Chapter 16.

The concept of intermittent pressure to prevent pressure sores was taken further by Keane (1979), who discussed the minimum physiological mobility requirement for man supported on a soft surface. Quoting from the work of Johnson *et al.* (1930), Laird (1935) and Oswald *et al.* (1963), he stated that the average interval between postural changes made during sleep by a normal adult subject was 11.6 minutes. He suggested therefore that 11.6 minutes is the minimum physiological mobility requirement (MPMR) to maintain the healthy state for short periods of soft-bed rest. He believed that when dealing with patients immobilised for long periods, as occurs following spinal injury, the optimum frequency of movement to prevent pressure damage of skin and muscle and impairment of physiological function of other organs was one gross postural change every 4.5 minutes. For this purpose he developed a turning bed, which provided automatic continuous turning of a patient from side to side through an excursion of 124 ° every 4.5 minutes. This equipment has been used since 1967 in certain centres worldwide. Great care must be exercised in immobilising the patient on the equipment to prevent him sliding from side to side during the 124° excursion, if shear damage of the tissues is to be avoided. The various laboratory and animal studies, coupled with the clinical reports of the use of ripple mattresses of one form or another and turning systems, suggest that intermittent pressures up to 50–100 mmHg (6.7–13.3 kPa) can be sustained by the tissues for 4 to 6 minutes without significant tissue damage. However, the movement of the tissues and the body caused by the various systems is not liked by some patients and the maintenance of the optimum environment at the patient–support interface is difficult to achieve.

As far back as 1873 it was realised that the prevention of potentially harmful distortion of the tissues could be achieved by floating the patient in water but separated from it by a loose waterproof sheet (Paget, 1873). This method of support, which provides hydrostatic or triaxial loading of the tissues, can be achieved only by using a fluid as the support medium. Fluids can be liquids, which are incompletely elastic and incompressible, or ideal gases, which are elastic and compressible. There is no solid support system, be it springs, rubber or plastics foam, that can provide the ideal support system for the severely disabled patient confined to bed with loss of pain sensation or musculoskeletal activity. In 1962 a prototype water immersion bed was constructed in which a very thin, loose plasticised polyvinyl chloride film was used to separate the patient from the water (Grant, 1967). The pressure applied to the body was directly proportional to the depth to which the body sank into the liquid and in the case of the buttock was approximately 23 mmHg (3.0 kPa). This pressure is normally below capillary pressure. The advantage of the system is that distortion of tissues is largely prevented and thus the continuously applied pressure has little effect on either the vascular or the lymphatic system. However, with this fluid system, evaporation of water vapour from the supported surface cannot occur. The instability of the support provided is not appreciated by the patient and nursing procedures are difficult, particularly with respect to lifting and positioning a patient.

Two gas support systems have been developed that enable the supine patient to be supported using pressures below normal capillary pressure. In one system, the LALBS (low air loss bed system) (Scales and Hopkins, 1971), temperature-controlled air is contained in 21 water-vapour-permeable but waterproof sacs. When the patient is correctly supported, the sacs deform and allow pressures below those which would cause capillary closure to be applied in a hydrostatic manner over the maximum surface area of the body (Krouskop *et al.*, 1984). The risk of urinary and circulatory complications can be prevented by adjusting the contour and attitude of the support system.

The development of an air fluidised bed was reported by Hargest and Artz in 1969. With this system of patient support some 40 cubic feet (1.13 cubic metres) per minute of temperature-controlled air is forced through a diffuser into a mass of soda–lime glass spheres in the size range 75–100 μm. The mass of spheres, approximately 30 mm in depth, is contained in the chamber or bed by a loose polyester filter sheet having a pore size of about 30 μm. The mass of glass spheres assumes the characteristics of a fluid and has a density of 2.0 compared with water and thus the patient floats on the bed rather than is contained in it. This bed is particularly useful for nursing patients with burn injuries in which the exposure method of treatment is used. However, in contrast to the LALBS, it is not possible to change the contour or attitude of the patient except by the use of pillows, since the glass spheres are subject to the effects of gravity. Both systems keep the skin dry and enable the skin temperature to be maintained at the optimum level, thus not increasing the metabolic demand in the tissues.

REFERENCES

Bader, D. L. and Bowker, P. (1983). Mechanical characteristics of skin and underlying tissues *in vivo*. *Biomaterials*, **4**, 305–308

Bader, D. L., Barnhill, R. L. and Ryan, T. J. (1986). Effect of externally applied skin surface forces on tissue vasculature. *Arch. Phys. Med. Rehabil.*, **67**, 807–811

Bennett, L., Kavner, D., Lee, B. K. and Trainor, F. A. (1979). Shear vs pressure as causative factors in skin blood flow occlusion. *Arch. Phys. Med. Rehabil.*, **60**, 309–314

Brown-Séquard, C.-E. (1852). Experimental researches applied to physiology and pathology. *Medical Examiner (Philadelphia)*, **8**, 481–504

Cattell, M. (1936). Physiological effects of pressure. *Biol. Rev.*, **11**, 441–476

Cochran, G. van B. (1979). Identification and control of biophysical factors responsible for soft tissue breakdown. Unpublished R.S.A. Progress Report, P.59173/2, No. 23

Daly, C. H., Chimoskey, J. E., Holloway, G. A. and Kennedy, D. (1976). Effect of pressure loading on the blood flow rate in human skin. In Kenedi, R. M., Cowden, J. M. and Scales, J. T. (eds), *Bed Sore Biomechanics*, Macmillan Press, London and Basingstoke, pp. 69–77

Exton-Smith, A. N., Overstall, P. W., Wedgwood, J. and Wallace, G. (1982). Use of the 'air wave system' to prevent pressure sores in hospital. *Lancet*, 5 June, **i**, 1288–1290

Gardner, W. J. and Anderson, R. M. (1948). Alternating pressure alleviates bedsores. *Mod. Hosp.*, **71** (5), 72–73

Grant, W. Russell (1967). Weightlessness in the treatment of bedsores and burns. *Proc. R. Soc. Med.*, **60**, 711–715

Groth, K.-E. (1942). Clinical observations and experimental studies on the origin of decubiti. *Acta. Chir. Scand.*, **87**, Suppl. 76: I, 1–209

Guttmann, L. (1953). The treatment and rehabilitation of patients with injuries of the spinal cord. In Cope, Z. (ed.), *Medical History of the Second World War, Surgery*, Vol. 2, HMSO, London, pp. 422–516

Hargest, T. S. and Artz, C. P. (1969). A new concept in patient care: The air fluidized bed. *A.O.R.N. J.*, September, **10**, 50–53

Hickman, V. E., Lindan, O., Reswick, J. B. and Scanlan, R. H. (1966). Deformation and flow in compressed skin tissues. In *Biomedical Fluid Symposium Proceedings*, Fluid Engineering Conference, American Society of Mechanical Engineers, 25–27 April 1967, pp. 121–147

Husain, T. (1953). An experimental study of some pressure effects on tissue with reference to the bed sore problem. *J. Path. Bact.*, **66**, 347–358

Jarrett, A. (1973). In *Physiology and Pathophysiology of the Skin*. Academic Press, New York, Chapter 8, pp. 267–294

Johnson, H. M., Swan, T. H. and Wiegand, G. E. (1930). In what positions do healthy people sleep? *J. Am. Med. Ass.*, **94** (26), 2058–2062

Jordan, M. M., Nicol, S. M. and Melrose, A. L. (1977). *Incidence of Pressure Sores in the Patient Community of the Borders Health Board Area on 13 October 1976*. University of Strathclyde Bioengineering Unit and Borders Health Board, Glasgow

Keane, F. X. (1979). The minimum physiological mobility requirement for man supported on a soft surface. Annual Scientific Meeting, International Society of Paraplegia, *Paraplegia*, **16**, 383–389

Kosiak, M. (1959). Etiology and pathology of ischaemic ulcers. *Arch. Phys. Med. Rehab.*, **40**, 62–69

Krouskop, T. A., Reddy, N. P., Spencer, W. A. and Secor, J. W. (1978). Mechanisms of decubitus ulcer formation – an hypothesis. *Med. Hypotheses*, **4** (1), 37–39

Krouskop, T. A., Williams, R. and Krebs, M. (1984). Effectiveness of air flotation beds. *Care, Science and Practice*, **4** (2), 9–11

Laird, D. A. (1935). Did you sleep well? *Rev. Rev.*, **91**, 23, 86, 321

Munro, D. (1940). Care of the back following spinal-cord injuries: A consideration of bed sores. *New Engl. J. Med.*, **223** (11), 391–398

Oswald, J. (1963). Melancholia and barbiturates: a controlled E.E.G. body and eye movement study of sleep. *Br. J. Psychiatry*, **100**, 66–78

Paget, Sir James (1873). Clinical lecture on bed-sores. *Students' J. and Hospital Gazette*, 10 May, **i**, 144–146

Palmer, J. D. K., Burke, G. E., O'Leary, J. P., Freed, M. and Krusen, F. H. (1968). Ulcer formation: Role of pressure and shear. *5th International Congress of Physical Medicine*, Montreal

Petersen, N. C. and Bittman, S. (1971). Epidemiology of pressure sores. *Scand. J. Plast. Reconstr. Surg.*, **5**, 62–66

Reddy, N. P., Cochran, G. van B. and Krouskop, T. A. (1981). Interstitial fluid flow as a factor in decubitus ulcer formation. *J. Biomechanics*, **14**, 879–881

Salmon, M.-M. (1936). *Arteries of the skin*. G. Masson et Cie, Paris. English translation Taylor, G. I. and Tempest, M. (eds), Churchill-Livingstone, Edinburgh, 1988, pp. 1–234

Scales, J. T. and Hopkins, L. A. (1971). Patient-support system using low-pressure air. *Lancet*, 23 October, **ii**, 885–888

Scales, J. T., Lowthian, P. T., Poole, A. G. and Ludman, W. R. (1982). 'Vaperm' patient-support system: a new general purpose hospital mattress *Lancet*, 20 November, **ii**, 1150–1152

Trumble, H. C. (1930). The skin tolerance for pressure and pressure sores. *Med. J. Aust.*, November, **ii**, 724–726

Vogel, H. G. (1977). Strain of rat skin at constant loads: influence of age and desmotropic agents. *Gerontology*, **23**, 77–86

Young, J. S. and Burns, P. E. (1982). Pressure sores and the spinal cord injured. In Young, J. S., Burns, P. E., Bowen, A. M. and McCutcheon, R. *Spinal Cord Injury Statistics: Experience of the Regional Spinal Cord Injury Systems*, Good Samaritan Medical Centre, Phoenix, Arizona, pp. 95–121

3

Pressure Sores: Clinical Aspects of Their Cost, Causation, and Prevention*

Brian Livesley

AN EXPENSIVE EPIDEMIC

Pressure sores are a recognised problem in hospitals, not only in the United Kingdom (Barbenel *et al.*, 1977; Lowthian, 1979; Roberts and Goldstone, 1979; Hibbs, 1982; Wright *et al.*, 1986) but also in countries as far apart as North America (Rubin *et al.*, 1974; Gerson, 1975; Walldorf, 1976; Robinson *et al.*, 1978; Allman *et al.*, 1986), Australia (Childs and Rimmington, 1983), South Africa (Manley, 1978) and Scandinavia (Petersen and Bittman, 1971; Ek and Bowman, 1982). The frequency with which they have been recorded in hospitals ranges from 2.7 to 66 per cent, with the highest figures occurring in aged patients with fractured femurs (Roberts and Goldstone, 1979; Versluysen, 1986).

In the United Kingdom, the cost of pressure sore care has been estimated to have risen from £60 million in 1973 (Editorial, 1973) to £150 million in 1982 (Scales *et al.*, 1982). This is equivalent to taking £750 000 out of the annual budget of every health district.

Other countries have also been making their own estimates. In Canada (Robinson *et al.*, 1978), pressure sore care for only four patients was calculated as costing $218 689 in 1976 and this had risen by 60 per cent (to $349 379) by 1977. The cost for 28 patients treated for pressure sores in the same Canadian hospitals was $652 148 and $1 million for 1976 and 1977 respectively. Similarly, in South Africa (Manley, 1978), a conservative estimate of pressure sore costs (made in 1976 for Cape Province at the Groote Schuur Hospital) was £1 300 000 in an area where there were 13 840 beds. More recently, and in the United States (Allman *et al.*, 1986), the cost of care increased the average charge of patient care from $7000 to $37 000 for those with pressure sores.

The general and local factors predisposing to, precipitating, and aggravating pressure sore development are described below – but what are the prime principles that need to be pursued to tackle this expensive epidemic,

---

*This chapter is reproduced by kind permission of *Nursing Times* from invited articles which first appeared on 6 August 1986 and 18 February 1987.

which hides beneath the bedclothes at home (Barbenel *et al.*, 1977; Petersen and Bittman, 1971; Hibbert, 1980) as well as in hospital? Prevention is obviously the keynote and requires prompt identification of patients at risk, with reduced periods spent lying on inappropriate surfaces, and the earliest positive management of those affected.

While several rating scales (notably the Norton (Exton-Smith *et al.*, 1982), Knoll (McFarlane and Castledine, 1982), and Waterlow (Waterlow, 1985) scheme) have been recommended to identify patients at risk, none has proved generally satisfactory (see Chapter 5). Patients aged over 65 years are at greatest risk and the importance of low-pressure patient support systems for elderly patients, from the point of entry to hospital until adequate mobility has been restored, has been well shown (Versluysen, 1986).

The next stage is, of course, to accept and act on the basis that this is not simply a nursing problem but also requires a planned and co-ordinated approach by clinicians and administrators. The latter must be more willing to release funds for the planned and cost-effective purchase of pressure-relieving mattresses and beds, now available as part of the new technology (Scales *et al.*, 1982; Exton-Smith *et al.*, 1982; Beaver, 1986).

Although improved use of the nursing process can go a long way to enabling every ward and hospital to produce its own information for analysis and action, two other issues are hindering this development. First, there is a widespread shortage of nursing staff, which is repeatedly highlighted by seasonal factors. Second, and according to one author (Jones, 1986), many nurses now in clinical practice have a great deal of knowledge about the nursing process but little experience and skill in using it to bring about solutions to patient problems in an organised, systematic, and efficient manner. National guidelines are now required. One other question, however, remains to be answered, 'Is there a failure to implement relevant nurse research findings at the bedside?' (Gould, 1985). To this author's eye a simple answer here is, 'Yes.' Certainly, there is tremendous scope for the development of the nurse specialist and ultimately the nurse consultant role to guide and direct relevant nursing research and to ensure its appropriate implementation.

PRACTICAL MANAGEMENT AND PREDISPOSING MEDICAL CONDITIONS

The importance of correct pressure area management is now beyond dispute. Indeed, even if we put to one side the severe discomfort and anxiety experienced by affected patients, the actual size and financial cost of the problem to the National Health Service in the United Kingdom is more than sufficient to demand our attention.

Since most people sleep for many hours each night in their own beds at home without developing pressure sores, it is pertinent to ask why they develop pressure sores in hospital, why some are more at risk than others, and what, if anything, can be done about it. As Versluysen says, 'Sores are not simply a ward or nursing problem, but an unintended consequence of hospital treatment' (Versluysen, 1986). Because of the ill-informed belief that they are merely the result of 'bad' nursing, pressure sores are commonly discussed in hushed tones as 'something we don't have in our hospital or my ward'. Despite the secrecy, because of embarrassment, the truth is that pressure sores affect 3–8.8 per cent of hospital patients (David, 1981). Indeed, in a large hospital admitting 100 patients daily, 5 patients will have developed pressure sores before the end of the first week.

The problem increases with the age of the patient and some patient groups are more at risk of developing pressure sores than others. Those with the highest risk of developing them are old people whose incontinence increases as they become bed- or chair-bound. Even within this age group, however, there are those more especially at risk. In a recent investigation of 100 elderly patients admitted consecutively to hospital with fracture of the femur, 66 developed sores and 83 per cent of these had developed them by day 5 in hospital (Versluysen, 1986).

Although as many as 21 variables have been used to predict pressure sore information with 98 per cent accuracy (Williams, 1972), both the Norton (Exton-Smith *et al.*, 1982) and the Knoll (McFarlane and Castledine, 1982) sore-risk rating scales are easier to use and have become well recognised by nurses as identifying patients who are most likely to develop at least one pressure sore. The problem, however, is not that simple. Several workers (Gosnell, 1973; Jones, 1980; Goldstone and Roberts, 1980; Pritchard, 1986) have found the need to develop their own pressure sore-risk scoring systems. In one case (Pritchard, 1986) this was because the Norton score was considered inadequate for assessing patients. But before we become confused by too many arbitrary scoring systems, we need to reconsider the basic principles involved in normal tissue perfusion and ask what goes wrong in ill people to lead to the formation of pressure sores.

In many patients, particularly the elderly, the foundations of intact and healthy pressure areas begin to erode once the patient becomes ill at home. The damage increases during prolonged waiting on a hard stretcher or treatment trolley pending investigation and ward transfer from the accident and emergency department. All nurses may be able to recall anecdotal instances of such prolonged waiting, but one study reveals that more than half of 86 elderly patients with fractured femurs spent over 3 hours on high-pressure surfaces before leaving the casualty department (Versluysen, 1986). What happens to the tissues in pressure areas during this wait, and why and how do pressure sores develop?

To appreciate what happens when pressure deforms the body surface of a healthy person, we need to understand what is meant by tissue stiffness. This can be described as the resistance to distortion present in the soft tissues of the body. You can demonstrate this by gently resting your thumb on the skin of your other forearm and then pressing the thumb down firmly. As you compress the skin, the fleshy parts of your forearm bulge away from the site of pressure. When you stop pressing, the site that was deformed by your thumb rebounds back to its normal position. This illustrates the resilient nature of healthy tissue.

If you repeat this simple experiment by pressing the back of your hand, you will note that the tissues are compressed between your thumb and the metacarpal bones. The pallor that occurs during the temporary occlusion of the blood vessels lasts longer than it did on the fleshy part of your forearm. This is because in the fleshy part of the forearm the tissue stiffness helps move the blood vessels away from the site of applied pressure. But, in the back of the hand, the blood vessels are not so free to move. They become trapped and compressed until they are bloodless between the pressing thumb and the resisting bone. These vessels then need time to refill after the applied pressure ceases.

If you now press firmly on the back of your hand for a full minute, you will note that on stopping, the skin beneath the thumbprint looks very pale and then gradually blushes with blood and becomes redder than the surrounding skin. This overfilling is due to reactive hyperaemia, a phenomenon discussed in detail in Chapter 12.

Normal tissue stiffness allows the body to resist deformation. The deeper blood vessels remain patent and blood flow continues. Persistent patency obviously depends upon where the balance lies between the tissue stiffness and intraluminal blood pressure, allowing the blood vessels to resist deformation (and occlusion) and the interface pressure applied to the body at the point of contact. If the interface pressure exceeds the summated values of the supporting tissue stiffness and the intraluminal blood pressure, the deeper blood vessels became bloodless and vice versa. Normally, the resting body can adjust to cope with the interface pressure arising from its weight. When tissue stiffness is reduced the body begins to sag. This sagging may result from several factors: for example, not only does dehydration reduce tissue stiffness, but during ageing there is a reduction in the number of elastic fibres which also increases the tendency of the aged body to sag. Thus tissue resilience is reduced. In addition at the site of an open sore, local sagging may become worse as tissue fluid seeps out of the body.

Tissue viability can be compromised further if blood flow to the areas at risk is:

1. flowing slower than normal because the patient has heart failure or a

reduced cardiac output because of atrial fibrillation or a recent myocardial infarction;
2. unable to carry sufficient oxygen because the patient is anaemic.

Once tissue viability is compromised, ischaemia leads first to deep tissue damage and then, by necrosis of the skin, to ulcer formation. Thus, a deep pressure sore is the result of tissue necrosis as a direct result of prolonged ischaemia following sustained compression of blood vessels. It is important to understand that in debilitated patients, who have impaired tissue stiffness and perfusion (for the reasons given below), a low pressure compressing the capillaries for long periods has a more serious effect on tissue viability than a high pressure compressing them for very short periods. Moreover, the development of low-pressure ischaemia gradually impairs nerve conduction and leads to local anaesthesia. Under these circumstances, even alert and articulate patients may be unaware that, for example, their heels are going gangrenous.

FACTORS PREDISPOSING TO PRESSURE SORES

These include:

a relatively immobile patient lying on a hard surface for prolonged periods;
areas of minimal soft tissue thickness where compression of the deeper
  blood vessels occurs against bony prominences. This explains why sacral,
  ischial and trochanteric areas, and also heels, are at high risk of
  developing pressure sores;
reduction of both tissue stiffness and the circulating blood volume by
  dehydration due to the following:
  low fluid intake, occurring readily in old people who have impaired thirst
    sensation and especially if they are confused or immobile;
  high fluid loss, including that from excessive diuretic therapy, diarrhoea
    and vomiting, acute blood loss, and uncontrolled diabetes;
  a pre-existing reduction in blood flow from cardiac pump failure, after
    myocardial infarction, acute atrial fibrillation, or in a drugged cardio-
    vascular system.

Once these predisposing factors are understood, the factors aggravating the formation of pressure sores can be seen in better perspective. These include general and local factors.

General Factors

These include anaemia (further reducing oxygen delivery to tissue which may already be ischaemic for the reasons given above) and previous malnutrition (making tissue breakdown and reduced repair more likely). Inappropriate sedation of the patient can produce immobility and predispose to pressure sore formation.

Local Factors

These include skin maceration by sweat, urine and faeces as well as damage from friction burns. This latter may be caused if the patient is moved, if the skin is dragged over a sheet, or, alternatively, if the skin is 'treated' by rubbing to 'protect' it. Fingerprint frictional tears in the skin surface may occur over the buttocks, especially when patients at risk of pressure sores are being turned over in bed by thoughtless hands. A variety of medicaments may produce local irritation and an allergic reaction predisposing to further skin breakdown. Another major local factor affecting pressure sore development is the type of dressing used on the sore, particularly in the early stages.

All of these general and local factors which can be relieved or prevented can lead to infection in the sore, which by promoting further necrosis and preventing healing may not only extend the sore but also predispose to the development of a life-threatening septicaemia.

RELIEVING PRESSURE

One way of reducing interface pressure is to use a pressure-relieving bed or mattress. This will not only reduce the direct pressure to the skin and subcutaneous tissues but also reduce the frictional shearing forces that would otherwise occur if a semi-recumbent patient slid down the bed. These direct and shearing factors produce both superficial damage and deep necrosis because of the compression of blood vessels.

Although many pressure-relieving systems have been devised, there have been very few properly *controlled* trials to demonstrate whether they are effective. One such trial on two alternating pressure devices compared the effectiveness of the large-cell Ripple mattress and the Pegasus airwave system in preventing and reducing the severity of pressure sores and promoting recovery from existing sores (Exton-Smith, 1982). The Pegasus system was found to be significantly more effective, more reliable, and free from mechanical breakdown. Other systems for reducing pressure include semi-automatic turning beds (viz. the net suspension bed, the Steeper

Mino CoRo, and the Stryker frame) and pressure-redistributing beds (viz. the water bed, the Clinitron bed, and the low-air-loss Mediscus bed).

Although pressure on areas can be relieved by turning the patient at regular intervals, this is commonly too time-consuming a procedure for wards which have a limited number of nurses and many dependent patients. *Indeed, with the modern bed technology now available, the tiring, regular manual turning of dependent patients by hard-pressed nurses attempting to prevent pressure sores should have become a practice of the past.* Such technology should not be accepted uncritically, however, but carefully evaluated so that the patient gains maximum benefit by being placed in the right bed!

REFERENCES

Allman, R. M., Laprade, C. A., Noel, L. B. *et al.* (1986). Pressure sores among hospitalised patients. *Ann. Intern. Med.*, **105**, 337–342

Barbenel, J. C., Jordan, M. M., Nicol, S. M. *et al.* (1977). Incidence of pressure sores in the greater Glasgow Health Board Area. *Lancet*, **2**, 548–550

Beaver, M. J. (1986). Mediscus low air-loss beds and prevention of decubitus ulcers. *Critical Care Nurse*, **6**, 5, 32, 33, 36–39

Childs, L. and Rimmington, P. M. (1983). Decubitus ulcers: a survey picture of two hospitals. *Austral. Nurses J.*, **13**, 1, 35–36

David, J. (1981). The size of the problem of pressure sores. *Care Science and Practice*, **1**, 10

Editorial. The costs of pressure on the patient (1973). *Lancet*, **2**, 309

Ek, A.-C. and Boman, G. A. (1982). A descriptive study of pressure sores; the prevalence of pressure sores and the characteristics of patients. *J. Advan. Nursing*, **7**, 51–57

Exton-Smith, A. N., Overstall, P. W., Wedgewood, J. and Wallace, G. (1982). Use of the 'Air Wave System' to prevent pressure sores in hospital. *Lancet*, **1**, 1288–1290

Gerson, L. W. (1975). The incidence of pressure sores in active treatment hospitals. *Internat. J. Nurs. Stud.*, **12**, 201–204

Goldstone, L. A. and Roberts, B. W. (1980). A preliminary discriminant function analysis of elderly orthopaedic patients who will or who will not contract a pressure sore. *Internat. J. Nurs. Stud.*, **17**, 17–23

Gosnell, D. J. (1973). An assessment tool to identify pressure sores. *Nursing Res.*, **22**, 55–59

Gould, D. (1985). Pressure for change. *Nursing Mirror*, **161**, 16, 28–30

Hibbert, D. L. (1980). A sore point at home. *Nursing Mirror*, **151**, 6, 40–41

Hibbs, P. (1982). Pressure sores: a system of prevention. *Nursing Mirror*, **155**, 5, 25–29

Jones, E. (1980). Prevention of Pressure Sores: The Clinical Sore Chart. *Nursing Times*, **76**, 565–566

Jones, J. (1986). An investigation of the diagnostic skills of nurses on an acute medical ward relating to the identification of risk of pressure sore development in patients. *Nursing Practice*, **1**, 257–267

Lowthian, P. (1979). Pressure sore prevalence: a survey of sores in orthopaedic patients. *Nursing Times*, **75**, 9, 358–360

Manley, M. T. (1978). Incidence, contributing factors and costs of pressure sores. *S. Afric. Med. J.*, **53**, 6, 217–222

McFarlane, J. and Castledine, G. (1982). *A Guide to the Practice of Nursing Using the Nursing Process*, Mosby, London, p. 39

Petersen, N. C. and Bittman, S. (1971). The epidemiology of pressure sores. *Scand. J. Plast. Reconstruct. Surg*, **5**, 62–66

Pritchard, V. (1986). Calculating the risk. *Nursing Times*, **82**, 8, 59–61

Roberts, B. V. and Goldstone, L. A. (1979). A survey of pressure sores in the over sixties on two orthopaedic wards. *Internat. J. Nurs. Stud.*, **16**, 355–364

Robinson, C. E., Coghlan, J. K. and Jackson, G. (1978). Decubitus ulcers in paraplegics: financial implications. *Canad. J. Pub. Hlth.*, **69**, 3, 199

Rubin, C. F., Dietz, R. R. and Abruzzese, R. S. (1974). Auditing the decubitus ulcer problem. *Amer. J. Nursing*, **74**, 1820–1821

Scales, J. T., Lowthian, P. T., Poole, A. G. *et al.* (1982). 'Vaperm' patient-support system: a new general purpose hospital mattress. *Lancet*, **2**, 1150–1152

Versluysen, M. (1986). How elderly patients with femoral fractures develop pressure sores in hospital. *Br. Med. J.*, **292**, 1311–1313

Walldorf, S. (1976). Significant changes in the care of patients with decubitii: how audit findings led to improved prevention and treatment protocols. *Quart. Rev. Bull.*, **2**, 11, 14, 15, 23, 24

Waterlow, J. (1985). A risk assessment card. *Nursing Times*, **81**, 49, 51–55

Williams, A. (1972). A study of factors contributing to skin breakdown. *Nursing Res.*, **21**, 238–243

Wright, D., Goodman, C. and Hall, D. (1986). Pressure to act. *Senior Nurse*, **59**, 1, 12–13

4

The Economics of Pressure Sore Prevention

Pam Hibbs

THE COST OF PRESSURE SORES

There are now increasing numbers of patients who survive serious illness or the multiple pathology of disease in old age and who are very much at risk in the development of pressure sores. There is indeed a serious epidemic but it remains a silent one hidden under the sheets.

The first aim of care must be in the prevention of pressure sores, as they are very serious for the patients who have them and they increase significantly the costs of health care. The resources available for health care are never going to be able to meet the demand. The economic scene has deteriorated owing to the recession, falling tax revenues from the private sector and the high cost of borrowing, as well as increases in raw-material prices beyond the general level of inflation. There is a need for good housekeeping now as never before. We need to be able to provide care of an appropriate quality and quantity at the lowest cost.

There is no exact total cost of pressure sores known as yet, although there have been many estimates made. The total cost was estimated in 1982 as in excess of £150 million (*Lancet*, 1982).

This could mean that each health district may well be spending £750 000 per year on this one condition. Unfortunately, our financial systems are not yet sophisticated enough for us to calculate individual patient costs, costs being usually aggregated for specialty budgets. It is also not clear if these estimates were the total costs of patients with pressure sores or the additional cost of healing the pressure sore alone. The patient with a pressure sore is often a very ill patient and may well represent a complex case. A patient with a penetrating pressure sore will need a prolonged hospital stay in order for the sore to be healed and for the patient's health to improve. This prolonged hospital stay will stop other patients using the bed, while for an elderly patient a long stay in hospital is particularly serious as they may lose their independence, rehabilitation will be delayed and then normal social networks of support may disappear, making it very difficult for them to return home.

When considering the economics of a pressure sore prevention programme it is worth remembering that it is not just the cost of treating

35

one patient's pressure sore during an extended stay that must be calculated, but also the benefits forgone by other patients who are denied care. Efficiency within health care can be described as making sure that the best output is obtained from the resource put in. To describe care as effective we need to know the standard set and also that the desired goals have been achieved.

There has been little systematic attempt to estimate the resource consequences of prevention. One study (Altman *et al.*, 1986) compared the total hospital charges at the Johns Hopkins Hospital for a sample of patients with sores ($W = 30$) and a sample of patients at risk of sores ($N = 78$). The reported ranges for hospital charges were large for the pressure sore group. Unfortunately, no study has yet been made of a large enough group of patients with pressure sores to determine the influence on the variables of each patient, and to decide whether the additional cost is due to the pressure sore or to the other complex pathology that the patient may suffer.

During a period of financial difficulty in 1987 it became necessary to justify the cost of a prevention programme. Although we all assumed that a patient who had developed a grade 4 pressure sore would be an expensive one, there was no definitive data available to prove the point. During this time a patient, 75 years of age, was transferred into St Bartholomew's Hospital with a complicated hip fracture and a gangrenous sacral pressure sore. From the time the patient was admitted the staff were asked to record all items and times of care for the whole of her stay. The total cost and the opportunity cost for 1987 are outlined as follows:

Direct Costs

Medical support	Standard cost × No. of days: £8.29 × 180	£1 492.00
Nursing support Qualified staff	Standard cost × No. of days: £25.24 × 180	4 543.00
Student nurse (3rd year)	Average cost × No. of days: £1.49 × 180	268.00
Radiographic support	Standard cost × No. of days: £2.892 × 180	507.60
Physiotherapy	Standard cost × No. of days: £2.46 × 180	442.80
Paramedical and diagnostic support	Standard cost × No. of days: £5.83 × 180	1 049.40
Carried forward		£8 302.80

Brought forward		£8 302.80
Medical and surgical supplies and equipment	Standard cost × No. of days: £7.47 × 180	1 344.60
Special bed hire	Weekly hire rate × No. of weeks plus delivery/installation and collection	
Clinitron Air Flotation Bed (9/52), SSI Medical Services, Nottingham		3 560.00
Pegasus Airwave System (13/52), Pegasus Airwave Ltd, Portsmouth		525.00
Non-pharmaceutical supplies	Item cost × No. of items utilised	
Silastic foam (10/52), Calmic Medical Division, Wellcome Foundation, Crewe	£81.16 × 2	162.32
Granflex dressing (8/52), Squibb Surgicare Ltd, Hounslow	£13.77 × 18	247.86
Pharmaceutical services and supplies	Standard cost × No. of days: £2.58 × 180	464.40
Special drugs	Average cost × No. of days: £3.21 × 180	577.80
Sugar paste (specially made)	Item cost × No. of items utilised: £21.60 × 2	43.20
Central sterile supply department	Standard cost × No. of days: £1.01 × 180	181.80
Operating theatre costs	Standard cost × No. of days: £14.65 × 180	2637.00
Miscellaneous direct services	Standard cost × No. of days: £0.79 × 180	142.20

Indirect Costs

'Overheads' – plus porterage, catering, cleaning, domestic services, plus lighting, heating, etc.	Standard cost × No. of days: £42.87 × 180	7 716.60
Total Cost		**£25 905.58**

Opportunity Costs

After looking at both the direct and the indirect costs incurred by treating an elderly orthopaedic patient with a grade 4 pressure sore, the opportunity costs should be considered. These have been defined by Knapp (1984) as:

The cost of using a resource in a particular service or mode of care is not the money cost or price of the resource, but is the benefit forgone (or opportunity lost) by losing its best alternative use.

Opportunity Cost: £25 905.58 per 180 days

Opportunity Costs – Alternative Estimates

The following examples illustrate the alternative ways of estimating the opportunity costs:

1. The standard cost per inpatient orthopaedic day costed in 1987 is £112.06. If this standard cost is divided into the aggregate cost of direct and indirect care and services for the patient with a grade 4 pressure sore, we arrive at the total number of standard inpatient days that could have been utilised, i.e.,

$$\frac{£25\,905.58}{£112.06} \quad \text{or} \quad \frac{\text{total direct and indirect costs}}{\text{standard cost per inpatient day}} = \frac{231 \text{ standard inpatient}}{\text{days}}$$

If we subtract the number of days that a patient with a grade 4 pressure sore utilised (180) from the standard inpatient days (231), we are left with 51 patient days that have been lost, or their use foregone, by other standard orthopaedic patients.

In other words, we have forgone the benefit of 51 extra (standard cost) inpatient days, which could have been put to alternative use.

2. The standard number of days per standard case is 10.9 days. If this standard time period is divided into the number of days that a grade 4 pressure sore patient utilises (180), we arrive at the standard number of cases that could have been treated had the bed not been occupied by 1 case. i.e.,

$$\frac{180}{10.9} \quad \text{or} \quad \frac{\text{number of days utilised by grade 4 patient}}{\text{standard no. of inpatient days}} = 17 \text{ standard cases}$$

Hence, the alternative usage of 1 patient's bed over a time span of 180 days could have increased throughout by 16 more cases, for example, hip or knee replacements, at an average case stay of 10.9 days. The foregone benefit that is denied us then is 169.1 standard patient days.

3.   The standard cost per 1 patient case is £1216.67: if this standard cost is divided into the aggregate cost of direct and indirect care, we arrive at the number of standard cases (per financial cost) that have been foregone, i.e.

$$\frac{£25\,905.58}{£1216.67} \quad \text{or} \quad \frac{\text{Aggregate cost of stay for grade 4 pressure sore patient}}{\text{standard cost per case}} = 21 \text{ standard cases}$$

Whereas the previous example shows the number of standard cases lost or foregone relative to time, this example shows the number of standard cases that have been lost (reduced throughput) in terms of comparative standard cost. The foregone benefit that is denied is 20 standard cases.

This detailed example was calculated from only one patient, but the financial arguments for investing in a pressure sore prevention programme appear convincing. Although our knowledge about pressure sores is advancing all the time, they have received little priority as a health care issue, despite the fact that with the increasing numbers of elderly people they are likely to become more frequent.

THE COST OF A PREVENTION PLAN FOR A HEALTH DISTRICT

Most pressure sores can be prevented if there is an active prevention plan known and implemented within the district. The elements of this prevention plan are as follows.

1.   *The Prediction of Patients Most Likely to Develop Pressure Sores*
There are many assessment tools, the best known of which is the Norton score (Norton *et al.*, 1962). Patients need to be identified as being at risk on admission and an individual plan of prevention made within one hour of admission. At present the external factors causing pressure sores are well known but the intrinsic factors are not so well understood. All tools are, therefore, fairly crude indicators. Many patients who are at risk do not go on to develop pressure sores. On the other hand, some patients who are not at risk according to the predictor will develop pressure sores. At the present time 25–30 per cent of the hospital- and community-nursed patients require a prevention plan; this number could be further reduced by having a more accurate predictor. Using predictors will not work on a once-only basis; use with very ill patients demonstrated that the score will vary. More efficient support systems may be required at different times in

the patient's illness. Patients who have permanent neurological damage
will require constant vigilance and support, but any intercurrent illness
such as an infection, or transfer to hospital or another care setting, will
require additional protection.

2. *Equipment Ideally Required for a Large Health District for Both Hospital and Community Patients in Any One Year*

Large-cell ripple beds, Talley Medical Equipment Ltd, Herts	300
Spenco silicore mattresses, Spenco (UK) Ltd, Steyning	400
Pegasus airwave beds, Pegasus Airwave Ltd, Portsmouth	60
Clinitron beds, SSI Medical Services, Nottingham	5
Fleeces, Brinmark Ltd, Coventry	600
Incubator pads, Spenco (UK) Ltd, Steyning	6
Wheelchair cushions (Roho), Raymar, Henley-on-Thomas	100

This equipment was not, of course, purchased all at the same time but was
a stock gradually built up over the years. There needs to be within the
organisation a system of assessing the need for new equipment to replace
that which has become old and outdated. This process should be in the
forward planning and budgetary planning of the organisation. The benefits
of prevention need to be demonstrated to management boards. It is also
not difficult to present a good case for the purchase and in-house
maintenance of some equipment rather than continually renting it.

A mattress replacement programme should be in operation; the continual use of the standard mattress distorts the foam and offers no
protection for vulnerable patients, as bottoming out can occur. This basic
piece of equipment is frequently overlooked and is used beyond its
working life in most hospitals. There should be a mattress renewal
programme ensuring that every mattress is renewed at least every 5 years.
It is also worth considering placing Vaperm mattresses (Mediscus, Ware-
ham) where there are more vulnerable patients, such as in the wards for
the elderly and in oncology and intensive-care units. These are more
expensive but will give greater comfort and protection and will reduce the
need for other support systems.

All pressure-relieving aids must be kept in good repair and available to
staff at the time of need, i.e. at any moment during the 24 hours, and each
district will therefore need to make maintenance arrangements for all
equipment to be cleaned and serviced.

Another reason for arguing for the economic benefits of a pressure sore
prevention programme and investing in efficient support systems that not
only will prevent pressure sores but will minimise the turning and lifting of
patients, is the health and wellbeing of the nurses and carers. For a long

time, pressure sores have been seen as a failure of nursing care. This is unfair. Research has indicated that poor equipment, delays in the process of care and lack of knowledge all contribute to their formation. Pressure sores also cause nurses guilt and distress as well as additional nursing work to perform. Heavy and very immobile patients will require an efficient support system for their own care and also to avoid the largest identifiable health hazard affecting nurses, namely, back injury. The greatest number of nurses' back injuries occurred in the medical, orthopaedic and geriatric wards (General, Municipal and Boilermakers Union, 1985). In their research, they found that in the course of 1 hour's work, two nurses in a geriatric ward lifted the equivalent of 2.5 tons weight. Community nurses are also at risk. Thus the provision of efficient hoists both for wards and for individual patients will do much to keep nurses healthy and at work as well as providing better care for the ill.

EDUCATION

For a successful plan of prevention, the cost of education for all members of the health care team is essential. All staff need to know how pressure sores develop and how delays of more than 1 hour in the process of care for susceptible individuals in all departments will contribute to this unwanted hazard of care. Staff need guidance and support. The appointment and cost of a specialist nurse who can become a useful source of expertise to staff will become cost effective and will lead to a decrease in the number of pressure sores. They can also initiate the different aspects of research and development, monitor the equipment used and make recommendations for individual problematic patients. Educating vulnerable patients who have a long-term problem and working with them to find their own plan of prevention that they can use everywhere is also very cost-effective. In addition we recommend the buying of equipment for the individual, which can be taken anywhere and which will hopefully reduce the incidence of pressure sores that occur when hospitalisation or intercurrent illnesses happen.

Information systems are essential in every health district that will monitor the incidence and severity of pressure sores occurring within the health care system. They can also be used to determine the most effective care and support systems used.

At the present time our financial systems are unable to systematically present us with an accurate estimate of the resource consequences of a prevention programme. As previously stated we need more accurate predictors to use and more evaluation of support systems, so that in the future it will be easier to identify the most cost-effective prevention systems. External factors causing pressure sores are well known, health authorities can be sued for allowing patients to develop pressure sores when it can be proven that an acceptable standard of care was not delivered. A health authority that offers no prevention steps to vulnerable patients will be in a poor position when litigation occurs. Recent awards have been in the region of £100 000 (Silver, 1987). Many patients such as these will make significant holes in a revenue budget. The resource consequences of prevention are only part of any evaluation of any prevention programme; even if prevention does not lead to a net saving in resources, it may still be justified in terms of the health benefits.

REFERENCES

Altman, R. M. *et al.* (1986). Pressure sores among hospitalised patients. *Annals of Internal Medicine*, **108**, 337–352

General, Municipal & Boilermakers Union (1985). *Hazard in the Health Service – An A–Z Guide Survey*, GMB, London

Knapp, M. (1984). *The Economics of Social Care*, Macmillan, London and Basingstoke

Lancet (1982). **2**, 1150–1152, The Cost of Pressure 150 million pounds

Norton, D., McLaren, R. and Exton-Smith, A. N. (1962). *Investigation of Geriatric Nursing Problems in Hospital*, National Corporation for the Care of Old People, London, reissued 1975, Churchill-Livingstone, Edinburgh

Silver, J. (1987). Letter. *Care, Science and Practice*, **5**, 30

5

Current Management for the Prevention of Pressure Sores

Rosemary A. Crow and Michael Clark

INTRODUCTION

The essence of prevention lies in identifying which patients are at risk of developing pressure sores, removing those factors which lead to tissue damage and monitoring progress of the patient's condition. Success requires some means of identifying vulnerable patients, counteracting the source of damage through matching vulnerability to methods of treatment and ensuring that the care provided remains effective. These aspects in combination form the basis of a strategy to ensure that good practice reaches all who require care.

IDENTIFYING THE RISK OF DEVELOPING PRESSURE SORES

In discussing the current methods available, it is important to recognise the distinction between identifying risk and assessing the nature of that risk. The former requires indicators predicting the development of pressure sores. The latter involves measurement of the responses of tissues under sustained loading, and recognition of aspects of the patient's condition which modify the body's mechanisms for coping with these applied loads.

The current techniques used to identify patients who are at risk are known collectively as 'risk calculators'. The earliest, and still probably the best-known, example is the Norton scale (Norton *et al.*, 1975). The patient's general physical condition, mental state, level of activity, level of mobility and incontinence are given a numerical score ranging from 1 to 4, with a final summation to give a 'Norton score'. The scale is detailed in Chapter 7 (see Table 7.1).

The lower the score, the higher the risk; the lowest total score that can be achieved is 5, the highest 20. Patients with a score of 14 or less are deemed to be those at risk and in need of pressure sore prevention (Norton, 1975).

Other risk calculators include those developed by Gosnell (1973; 1987)

43

and Waterlow (1985). Gosnell's scale is based on that of Norton, but instead of scoring physical condition it scores nutrition. The scale also reverses the scoring system, so that within the same range of 5 and 20 those at risk score highest. No specific cut-off point is identified. Waterlow's system scores build/weight for height, visual skin type at risk areas, continence, mobility, sex, age, appetite and a series of special risks such as poor nutrition, sensory deprivation, high-dose anti-inflammatory and steroid drugs, smoking more than 10 cigarettes a day, orthopaedic surgery and fracture below the waist. Scores are weighted according to assumed risk and several scores can be used in some of Waterlow's categories. Any patient with a score of 10 or more is deemed to be at risk; high and very high risk are reflected in scores of greater than 14 and 19 respectively.

Choice of Calculator

The choice of which risk calculator to use depends upon its suitability for the patients for whom care is being organised. The criteria which can be used to inform choice are: (1) accuracy in predicting those who are 'at risk'; (2) ease and convenience in use; and (3) reliability between staff and patients.

To be effective in predicting risk, the risk calculator needs to include measures which characterise vulnerability. For it to be of clinical value it should identify all who are 'at risk' without either over-inclusion, which could lead to misuse of expensive and scarce resources, or omission, which deprives of care those patients who need it.

Choice Based on Characteristics of Vulnerability

The patient groups in which sores are frequent are those over the age of 70 years, and those who suffer from multiple sclerosis, Parkinson's disease, cerebro-vascular disease resulting in paralysis, spinal-cord injury, fractured neck of femur, arthritis and rheumatism, diseases of the peripheral and central circulatory system and diabetes mellitus (Jordan and Clark, 1977; Young *et al.*, 1982; David *et al.*, 1983; Versluysen, 1986). Aspects of the patient's clinical condition said to be associated with the presence of pressure sores are reduced spontaneous body movement among elderly hospitalised patients in bed (Exton-Smith and Sherwin, 1961), protein deficiency in paraplegic and tetraplegic patients (Kermani *et al.*, 1970; Moolton, 1972) and lowered leucocytic ascorbic acid concentrations in paraplegic patients (Burr *et al.*, 1972). Other factors associated with the presence of a pressure sore are collagen breakdown in patients with a spinal-cord injury (Claus-Walker *et al.*, 1973), and altered collagen synthesis in elderly patients. Collagen synthesis may also be impaired through emotional stress owing to an increased circulation of glycocorticoids (Krouskop, 1983).

Vulnerability of skin and soft tissue is reflected in the response of skin blood flow under applied loads. The generally accepted limit of pressure which tissue can withstand has been considered to be below 32 mmHg (4.3 kPa). In reality, the response to loads varies between individuals (Bader and Gant, 1988; Bennett *et al.*, 1979; Ek *et al.*, 1987). Skin blood flow can cease in hemiplegic patients when external pressures of only 11 mmHg (1.5 kPa) are applied (Ek *et al.*, 1987). In some geriatric patients, flow can be occluded under external pressures as low as 20 mmHg (2.7 kPa), but in others flow was detected at pressures of 120 mmHg (16 kPa) (Bennett *et al.*, 1981).

Vulnerability is thus identifiable at three levels, as follows:

1. general categorisation according to age and medical condition;
2. presence of characteristics which describe the patient's general clinical condition (e.g., level of mobility, nutritional status, presence of anxiety);
3. specific measures of skin blood flow and its response to externally applied loads.

The Norton and Gosnell scales grade the *presence of characteristics* to arrive at a total care. Waterlow's scale, as well as grading *the presence of characteristics*, uses *general categories* such as age, medical condition, surgery and medication. None includes specific measures which would indicate tissue response to applied loads.

Choice Based on the Clinical Value of the Calculators

The Norton scale has been systematically tested for its ability to predict whether geriatric hospital patients or patients over the age of 60 admitted to hospital with a fractured neck or femur develop sores (Norton *et al.*, 1975; Goldstone and Goldstone, 1982). The study of geriatric hospital patients (Norton *et al.*, 1975) suggests that at the cut-off point of 14 some patients will be missed (21 per cent of patients who develop sores scored between 15 and 17 and 5 per cent between 18 and 20). Over-inclusion is also apparent; only 50 per cent of the patients with a score of less than 12 subsequently developed sores.

In the group of elderly orthopaedic patients (Goldstone and Goldstone, 1982), 89 per cent of patients who developed sores were identified as at risk, but this was at the expense of including 64 per cent of patients who did not subsequently develop sores. Within this group of patients the Norton scale casts its net widely in achieving a reasonable level of sensitivity. How reliably patients would be recognised by different staff or when assessment is repeated on the same patient was not reported in either study.

Waterlow's scale was assessed on a more heterogeneous group of 650 patients (Waterlow, 1985). All patients who developed sores scored over 12. No information is available on how many patients who scored over 12 *did not* develop sores, nor what the results were for patients who scored between 10 and 12. Repeatability of scores was not reported either.

Thus the Norton scale both over-predicts and may miss some vulnerable patients. Without more systematic testing, no conclusion can be reached about Waterlow's scale. All calculators are said to be quick and reasonably easy to administer but there is no information about their reliability. There are therefore no strong arguments to favour any one calculator except that only the uses and limitations of the Norton scale have really been systematically studied, and even then remain incomplete. But whichever one is chosen, the score arrived at merely indicates risk. Given the individual nature of tissue response to external loads, they miss an essential aspect, i.e. the need to measure the patient's tissue response to external pressure so that appropriate treatment which removes or counters the sources of danger can be selected. Further individual assessment is therefore required to establish the care required.

SELECTING TREATMENT TO PREVENT PRESSURE SORES

The purpose to treatment in prevention is to reduce the patient's vulnerability to tissue damage. Approaches include reducing damaging pressures on the skin, in addition to the clinical prescription which will improve the architecture and integrity of the tissue.

Reducing Damaging Loads

It is important to recognise the distinction between abrasions and sores which arise from necrosis of soft tissue. Abraded sores (grade 2 sores) arise following weakening or physical damage to the epidermis (David *et al.*, 1983). They are a result of friction between the skin and its support surfaces when these surfaces are in contact and move against each other. Sores which affect the dermis and muscle (grade 3 and 4 sores) result from horizontal or vertical loads which damage the integrity of the soft tissue, leading to necrosis.

Avoiding Friction

In the skin, anything which softens the tissue, such as contact with urine, or changes in the skin micro-climate, such as a raised skin temperature, increases the likelihood of damage from friction. Additionally, anything that increases the surface roughness or hardness of the support surface produces problems (Clark, 1985). Laundering techniques are thought to be a major contributory factor.

Treatment therefore includes the following:

1. Maintaining a dry interface between skin and its support surface; patients may require positive management of their continence.
2. Use of soft surfaces as covers where hard or rough surfaces cannot be avoided; sheepskins are suitable so long as they are large enough to cover the entire support surface, but their use may increase skin temperature.
3. Checking for evidence of abrasion and removing the source; common problems are legs or side arms of wheelchairs, ill-fitting prostheses, and ill-fitting shoes.

All patients identified as being 'at risk' are vulnerable to abrasion.

Reducing Pressure

Effects of pressure can be relieved either by its uniform redistribution or through its rhythmic elimination. Matching the appropriate support surface to individual requirements involves recognition of the susceptible sites and selection of equipment which reduces potentially dangerous levels of pressure.

The most vulnerable anatomical sites are those areas of tissue over bony prominences. But the relative risk of tissue damage depends upon the individual's position. *In bed*, when the individual is supine or lateral supine the sites at risk are the shoulder, sacrum, trochanter, heel and external malleolus. When supine, contact pressures are highest under the heels, but if the knees are bent pressures are highest at the sacrum (Ek *et al.*, 1987). When semi-recumbent, the sites at risk are the sacrum, ischial tuberosities and heels. *In sitting*, the principal sites at risk are at the ischial tuberosities. Contact pressure readings between 100 mmHg (13.3 kPa) and over 300 mmHg (40 kPa) have been recorded from healthy subjects seated on a flat surface (Treaster, 1987).

Support surfaces need to be selected on their performance in reducing applied pressures to levels which do not impede skin blood flow. Salisbury (1985) noted the difficulty in selecting single criteria upon which comparisons of the effectiveness of different support surfaces can be made. The problem is exemplified by the alternating pressure supports; should these be compared with the static systems when at their maximum, minimum or some intermediate pressure? The differences are illustrated in Figures 18.1–18.3.

Clark (1987) suggests that one parameter which can be used is pressure impulse, the total pressure which each system exerts over a fixed period of time. This he obtained by measuring interface pressure at the trochanter every 2 seconds for 15 minutes, and extrapolating from this to give a total pressure per bed hour. To set these total pressures within a framework categorising support effectiveness, known skin capillary and venous pressures, in conjunction with information about how external pressures are transmitted to deeper tissues (Le *et al.*, 1984), were used to compare a series of thresholds representing tissue vulnerability (Table 5.1) graded

Table 5.1 Patient support surface classification based upon the total pressure exerted per hour at the greater trochanter

Support surface category	Pressure impulse $(\times 10^{-4}\,mmHg\,h^{-1})$	Equivalent instantaneous pressure (mmHg)	% Measurement time at 0 mmHg
1	>8.46	>47	0
2	6.93–8.45	38.5–47.0	0
3	5.40–6.92	30.0–38.4	0
4	3.78–5.39	21.0–29.9	0
5	2.16–3.77	12.0–20.9	0
6	<2.16	<12	0
7	n.a.	n.a.	10–20*
8	n.a.	n.a.	>20*

*Based on Le *et al.* (1984).

from 1 (providing only low pressure relief) to 8 (providing complete relief). To illustrate this grading system, Clark (1987) provided total pressures allowing preliminary categorisations of some commonly available support systems in the United Kingdom as follows:

Grade 2 4.5-inch foam mattress (e.g. Vaperm); silicore-filled products (e.g. Spenco mattress)
Grade 3 Sheepskin on foam mattress
Grade 5 Correctly inflated single-deck alternating mattress (e.g. Talley large-cell ripple)
Grade 7 Double-layer alternating mattress (e.g. Pegasus airwave system)

It should be noted that these interim categorisations are based on samples of between 1 and 10 subjects, and are liable to reassessment when sample sizes are increased.

Based on this categorisation, foam and silicore mattresses (including the addition of sheepskins) are only suitable for low-risk patients. High-risk patients, on the other hand, require either single-deck or double alternating mattresses according to the degree of their vulnerability. Evidence from clinical trials shows that alternating-pressure mattresses reduce the incidence of pressure sores, particularly when double-layered (Exton-Smith *et al.*, 1982).

Heels are a particular problem on almost all the commonly used support surfaces and pressure will be increased by the weight of bedclothes. For all patients at risk it is advisable to lift the weight of bedclothes off the feet by either using a bed-cradle or using a duvet instead of sheets and blankets.

Scientific analysis of mattress supports is covered further in Chapter 18.

MONITORING THE PATIENT'S PROGRESS

The underlying purpose of monitoring progress is to ensure that care remains effective in combating vulnerability. The continuing management of prevention thus requires the following:

1. repeated assessment of the patient's vulnerability;
2. regular appraisal of changes in the response of the skin to external loads;
3. maintenance of support surfaces in efficient working order.

The key factors are repeated records of the previous measures, allowing comparison between the risk scores, and descriptions of the patient's general condition. In nursing, recommendations about care plans stress components concerned with a general nursing history, 'goals' of care, and the nursing prescription (Hunt and Marks-Maran, 1980). However, standardised records based on the concept of *nursing care plans* require additions to include repeated measures of the *patient's* condition if they are to be used for evaluating the *patient's* progress.

STRATEGY TO ENSURE GOOD PRACTICE

Planning a pressure sore prevention programme requires knowledge of the size and extent of the problem in order that adequate resources can be provided and any failures in the delivery of care identified.

Prevalence and Incidence of Pressure Sores

Figures upon which a strategy can be based are the prevalence and incidence rates of patients with sores. Results, however, do need to be interpreted in the light of the characteristics of the population studied. For example, from a national study (David *et al.*, 1983) the overall prevalence of hospital patients with pressure sores was shown to be 6.7 per cent. There was, however, considerable variation in prevalence between districts (ranging from 3.5 per cent to 10.8 per cent) and hospital wards (5.1 per cent to 16 per cent), with the highest individual rates being found on GP units (8.2 per cent) and geriatric (9.2 per cent), orthopaedic and trauma (7.7 per cent) and general medical wards (6.7 per cent).

Clearly, surveys used as a basis for planning care need to be carried out locally so that they provide information about the population for whom they service. Furthermore, the majority of published reports only 'include the hospital population. Study needs to be widened to include patients in the community and designed so that it covers groupings present in the organisation of local care, e.g. hospital ward, unit or department; community neighbourhoods or primary care groups. Areas found to have high prevalence rates can then be re-examined to identify the nature of the problem as Versluysen (1986) did by studying the *incidence* of sores in a group of elderly patients with a femoral fracture. The cause appeared to be related to the time the patient spends in the casualty department rather than to care in the orthopaedic ward (see Chapter 6).

Establishing Adequate Resources

An estimate of requirements can be based upon the size of the population judged to be 'at risk' from pressure sores, established by Hibbs as between 25 and 30 per cent of the hospital population.

If there is no inventory of equipment for the district, a survey of current stocks and their whereabouts carried out before the purchase and distribution of resources will inform discussion (Clark and Crow, 1988). Again, comparison of estimated resource needs between health districts requires caution. This is discussed in Chapter 4, where Hibbs recommends a list of equipment, basing her estimation for the City and Hackney Health Authority on a wider hospital population which included community requirements.

Assuring Good Practice

An important component of any strategy is maintaining the standard of care. Studies have shown that not all nurses use a screening device to detect patients 'at risk', even though they know of the availability of appropriate tools (Wright and Goodman, 1985; Gould, 1986). Even when risk calculators are used, there is a suggestion from Abruzzese (1982) that no more care is provided. A critical factor is thus ensuring that knowledge is translated into practice.

Reports suggest that a regular review of the prevalence rates is a means of keeping the numbers of patients with sores low (Gosnell, 1987; Hibbs, 1987). Providing guidelines for good practice gives further support and, if targets are reviewed periodically, a way of maintaining awareness. The Royal College of Physicians of England in their report on physical disability (1986) recommend that every district health authority should have a pressure sore service which includes a regular survey of prevalence and incidence of pressure sores, a readily available supply of essential equipment, a written district policy covering prevention and management and a designated senior member of both the medical and nursing staff with responsibility for running the service.

REFERENCES

Abruzzese, R. S. (1982). *The Effectiveness of an Assessment Tool in Specifying.* Adelphi Report, *Nursing Care to prevent Decubitus Ulcers.* In Holt, J. and Woog, P. (eds), PRN: The Adelphi Report 1981–82, Adelphi University, New York, 1982

Bader, D. L. and Gant, C. A. (1988). Changes in transcutaneous oxygen tension as a result of prolonged pressures at the sacrum. *Clin. Phys. Physiol. Meas.*, **9**, 33–40

Bennett, L., Kavner, D., Lee, B. Y. and Trainor, F. S. (1979). Shear vs pressure as causative factors in skin blood flow occlusion. *Arch. Phys. Med. Rehab.*, **60**, 309–314

Bennett, L., Larner, D., Lee, B. Y., Trainor, F. S. and Lewis, J. H. (1981). Skin blood flow in seated geriatric subjects. *Arch. Phys. Med. Rehab.*, **62**, 392–398

Burr, R. G. and Rajan, K. T. (1972). Leucocytic ascorbic acid and pressure sores in paraplegia. *Br. J. Nutrition*, **28**, 275–281

Clark, M. (1985). Farrowing pen floor abrasiveness measured using a rubber-block drag test. *Farm Building Progress*, **80**, 29–32

Clark, M. (1987). Continuous interface pressure measurement using an electro-pneumatic sensor: The SCP monitor. *Care Science and Practice*, **5**(2), 5–8

Clark, M. and Crow, R. (1988) *Pressure Sores and the Provision of Pressure-Relieving Aids and Appliances Across Four Hospitals in S. W. Surrey District Health Authority.* Report to S. W. Surrey District Health Authority, University of Surrey, Guildford

Claus-Walker, J., Campos, R. J., Carter, R. E. and Chapman, M. (1973). Electrolytes in urinary calculi and urine of patients with spinal cord injuries. *Arch. Phys. Med. Rehab.*, **54**, 109–114

David, J. A., Chapman, R. G., Chapman, F. J. and Lockett, B. (1983). *An Investigation of the Current Methods Used in Nursing for the Care of Patients with Established Pressure Sores.* Nursing Practice Research Unit, University of Surrey, Guildford

Ek, A. C., Gustavssen, G. and Lewis, D. H. (1987). Skin blood flow in relation to external pressure and temperature in the supine position on a standard hospital mattress. *Scand. J. Rehab. Med.*, **19**, 121–126

Exton-Smith, A. N. and Sherwin, R. W. (1961). The prevention of pressure sores: The significance of spontaneous bodily movements. *Lancet*, **ii**, 1124–1126

Exton-Smith, A. N., Overstall, P. W., Wedgewood, J. and Wallace, G. (1982). Use of the 'air wave system' to prevent pressure sores in hospital. *Lancet*, **i**, 1288–1290

Goldstone, L. A. and Goldstone, J. (1982). The Norton Score: an early warning of pressure sores? *J. Adv. Nursing*. **7**, 419–426

Gosnell, D. (1973). An assessment tool to identify pressure sores. *Nursing Research*, **22**, 55–59

Gosnell, D. (1987) Assessment and evaluation of pressure sores. *N. Clinics of North America*, **22**, 399–416

Gould, D. (1986). Pressure prevention and treatment: an example of nurses' failure to implement research findings. *J. Adv. Nursing*, **1**(4), 389–394

Hibbs, P. (1987). 22 Clinical features; preventing an 'unnecessary evil'. *Nursing Standard, December*

Hunt, J. and Marks-Maran, D. J. (1980). *Nursing Care Plans*. H.M.&M. Publishers, Aylesbury

Jordan, M. M. and Clark, M. O. (1977). *Report on the Incidence of Pressure Sores in the Patient Community of the Greater Glasgow Health Board Area on the 21 January 1976*. The Bioengineering Unit, University of Strathclyde and the Borders Health Board, University of Strathclyde, Glasgow

Kermani, S. R., Siddique, M., Zain, S. and Kazi, K. (1970). Biochemical studies on pressure sore healing in paraplegics. *Paraplegia*, **8**, 36–41

Krouskop, T. A. (1983). A synthesis of the factors that contribute to pressure sore formation. *Medical Hypothesis*, **11**, 255–267

Le, K. M., Madsen, B. L., Barth, P. W., Ksander, A. M., Angell, J. B. and Vistnes, L. M. (1984). An in-depth look at pressure sores using monolithic silicon pressure sensors. *Plast. Reconstruc. Surg.*, **74** (6), 745–754

Moolton, S. E. (1972). Bedsores in the chronically ill. *Arch. Phys. Med. Rehab.*, **53**, 430–438

Norton, D. (1975). Research and the problem of pressure sores. *Nursing Mirror*, February, 65–67

Norton, D., McLaren, R. and Exton-Smith, A. N. (1975). *An Investigation of Geriatric Nursing Problems in Hospital*. Churchill-Livingstone, Edinburgh

Royal College of Physicians (1986). Physical disability in 1986 and beyond. A report of the Royal College of Physicians. *J. R. Coll. Phys. Lond.*, **20** (3), 160–194

Salisbury, R. E. (1985). Transcutaneous PO_2 monitoring in bed-ridden burn patients: a physiological analysis of four methods to prevent pressure sores. In Lee, B. Y. (ed.), *Chronic Ulcers of the Skin*, McGraw-Hill, New York, pp. 189–196

Treaster, D. (1987). Measurement of Seat Pressure Distributions. *Human Factors*, **29** (5), 563–575.

Versluysen, M. (1986). How elderly patients with femoral fracture develop pressure sores in hospital. *Br. Med. J.*, **292**, 1311–1313

Waterlow, J. (1985). A risk assessment card. *Nursing Times*, **49**, 51, 55

Wright, D. and Goodman, C. (1985). *Pressure Sore Study Newsletters*. Reports from the Community Medicine and Nursing Research Unit, St Mary's Hospital, Paddington, London

Young, J. S., Burns, P. E., Bowen, A. M. *et al.* (1982). *Spinal Cord Injury Statistics: Experience of the Regional Spinal Cord Injury System*, Good Samaritan Medical Centre, Phoenix, Arizona, pp. 85–121

Part II
Experiences in Various Clinical Disciplines

6

Orthopaedics

Christopher Bulstrode

INTRODUCTION

The incidence of pressure sores in orthopaedics is probably higher than in any other practice. This includes the problems of the paraplegic patient, whose care may fall to the orthopaedic surgeon but who presents special problems which are dealt with in another chapter. Even excluding these patients, it seems likely that more pressure sores in Britain are associated with an orthopaedic admission than with any other factor. This reflects the fact that many of the patients admitted to orthopaedic units either already have or are at high risk of developing pressure sores. There is also a direct association between some surgical practices and pressure sores.

In this chapter I will discuss some of these factors and what may be done to reduce the number of pressure sores to a minimum.

PRESENT ATTITUDES

There are units in this country which still regard pressure sores as an integral part of an orthopaedic practice, an unfortunate but necessary evil. It is certainly true that it may be well-nigh impossible to eradicate pressure sores completely, and that constant vigilance is necessary to hold levels to a minimum, but pressure sores are not integral to the practice. Other units may claim that they *never* have pressure sores. It is my experience that in those units where this claim is made there are *always* pressure sores present and that the claim represents a failure in monitoring, not an excellence of care. Honest monitoring is important, and each time a new pressure sore is discovered it should pose the questions, 'Has there been a failure in the care of the patient at some stage? If so, how can this be avoided in future?'

INCIDENCE

The incidence of pressure sores in orthopaedic practice is not clearly known, despite the fact that many units keep a careful record of the number of patients with sores in a register of pressure sores. There is however comparable data to show that pressure sores in orthopaedic units are more common than in other in-patient units. Jordan (1977a, b) has published figures for the incidence in orthopaedic units and a further similar study for those in all in-patients in the same district (Sheppeard *et al.*, 1980, Versluysen 1985). The figures given are 12 per cent and 19 per cent incidence for orthopaedic wards and around 9 per cent for all in-patients. Within orthopaedic units the incidence in the literature varies from 2.7 per cent (Lienbach and Barlow, 1973) in a purely elective orthopaedic practice to 42.7 per cent (Ferris, 1983) in a sample consisting only of trauma cases. My own unpublished experience in a hospital, now closed, was of a maximum incidence of just under 75 per cent in a mainly trauma unit, with an incidence of around 30–50 per cent at other times. The large range of percentages is in part a result of differing types of orthopaedic practice, elective orthopaedics having a lower incidence than traumatic. Figures from the Royal National Orthopaedic Hospital (Lowthian, 1979), gathered in 1978, when only a small proportion of the patients were trauma admissions, revealed an incidence of only 7 per cent. However, a paper discussing the complications of internal fixation of femoral fractures (trauma) from Exeter gives an incidence of pressure sores between 2 and 6 per cent (Heyse-Moore *et al.*, 1983), while a paper discussing the complications of elective total hip replacement from Oswestry gives a 21 per cent incidence of pressure sores (Sheppeard *et al.*, 1980). A more normal mix of patients in a standard orthopaedic unit is given by Versluysen (1985), where 63 per cent of the patients were undergoing surgical treatment for traumatic fractured neck of femur, while 17 per cent were admitted for elective total hip replacement. The incidence in this paper is 32 per cent overall, but 92 per cent of the pressure sores were in the patients with a fractured neck of femur, giving an incidence of 38 per cent for trauma and only 14 per cent in elective cases.

Pressure sores are also more common in older patients. Versluysen's data records no pressure sores in patients under 60 years of age. Among those patients aged between 60 and 70, it was 30 per cent, while in patients over 70 it was just under 50 per cent. She also demonstrated that despite the higher incidence of female admissions than male, the incidence of sores in females was twice that of males. However, it is not possible from her data to correct for the difference in age of admission between male and female. It may therefore be that this effect is the result of age differences on admission rather than a true sexual dimorphism.

The time of onset of pressure sores during an admission is an emotive problem, there being a temptation to justify the presence of a pressure sore by stating that it was present before admission. As I shall discuss later in this chapter, there are good theoretical reasons to believe that the trauma leading to sore formation may well occur quite commonly before admission to hospital. Versluysen's data supports this possibility: 17 per cent of the sores were present on admission, while 34 per cent developed sores within the first week and a further 24 per cent in the second week. Surgery itself is again a potent cause of pressure sores. In Versluysen's data 18 per cent had a sore before operation, while 16 per cent developed a sore on the actual day of operation, 34 per cent in the week after surgery and only 13 per cent in the second week after surgery. The day of surgery appears to be the single most important period for sores to develop. It is not clear how variable the interval may be between insult to the soft tissues and the first record of a grade 2 pressure sore. This clearly depends both on the vigilance of the staff and on the actual pathological course of the necrosis and may further complicate the picture recorded in the various papers.

Despite these rather confusing features, some conclusions can be drawn. This does suggest that pressure sores are indeed found more commonly on orthopaedic wards than elsewhere. Versluysen provides the only data where the incidence between trauma and elective cases can be compared and the incidence differs by a factor of more than 2, sores being more common in trauma patients than elective ones.

CAUSATION

The causation of pressure sores in orthopaedic practice is multi-factorial in terms of both the mechanism involved and the clinical responsibility for occurrence. This may well go some way to explain why so little has been achieved in some units in terms of reducing the morbidity from the condition and why other units have been so successful. In this section it seems logical to go through an admission for fractured neck of femur and analyse risk factors at each stage of the admission.

Admission for Fractured Neck of Femur: Risk Periods

The Fall

There is a marked increase in the number of elderly in the population. The association with fractured neck of femur and the elderly has led to what verges on an epidemic of fractured neck of femur patients over the past few years (Duthie, 1981). The commendable efforts of the Health Service in trying to care for the elderly in the community rather than within institutions has inevitably led to large numbers of the elderly living at home who are only just able to cope. Supervision may be minimal, or in many cases completely absent. A fall under these circumstances may result in the patient spending some time on the floor unable to move before help finally arrives. During this time on the floor patients may inevitably lie in one position on a hard floor. Furthermore they may become hypothermic and dehydrated, two further factors which may reduce the soft tissue's resistance to breakdown and lead to the formation of a pressure sore. These sores may not be noted on admission to hospital, firstly because no one trained and alert to the problems of pressure sores assesses the patient in the reception area. Secondly, the necrosis caused by the patient's enforced immobility on the floor may only be manifest as a slight reddening of the affected area (grade 1 sore). It is only later that the inevitable progression to a fully developed sore will become obvious. It is therefore clear that the patients making up the current epidemic of fractured neck of femur both belong to an age group at high risk of developing pressure sores and may indeed have already been exposed to conditions adequate for their creation before the ambulance has even been called.

Transport

The transport of severely dehydrated patients must always be performed with the utmost caution, as even a small amount of movement in a stretcher or the firm grip needed to lift a patient may cause tissue breakdown. I have never seen a pressure sore caused by ambulance transport in this country, as crews are trained to a very high standard in the care of patients, but in rescue services under difficult conditions (such as mountain rescue) this can be an important problem. Air splints provide a further problem. Local pressure in excess of 60 mmHg can be obtained from the creases in a fully inflated splint (D. L. Bader, personal communication). Unless great care is taken to ensure that pressures are kept low and that the splint is deflated for at least 10 minutes every hour, pressure sores may result.

Accident and Emergency Department

There are considerable problems for an elderly trauma patient in an accident and emergency department. Because on the whole they are quiet and uncomplaining patients, they receive relatively low priority in an accident service swamped with work, staffed by inexperienced doctors and geared to processing patients on priority. Patients with a suspected fractured neck of femur are placed on an X-ray trolley which is both hard and narrow. It is difficult and dangerous to turn such a patient while they remain on a trolley. However, before they can be transferred into a bed the following events must occur.

1. Details are taken by the receptionist.
2. The patient is then assessed by sister and put into a bay where they are undressed and examined by a nurse.

3. They are then seen by a doctor, examined and routine investigations performed. This will include an ECG and some X-rays.
4. For the X-rays they must be transferred into another department and wait in another queue for this examination.
5. They then return to the accident service and wait again to be seen by the doctor.
6. Arrangements are then made for their transfer to a ward. It may take some time to find an available bed ready to receive the patient.
7. Further delays may then occur before the porters and nurse are available to make the transfer to a ward.

It is difficult to measure the time involved in this complex procedure of taking a patient from the ambulance stretcher to a hospital bed, as observation of the details inevitably leads to the patient receiving preferential treatment. However, the time period has never in my experience been less than 1 hour and in many cases exceeds 6 hours during busy periods in the accident service. These figures were gathered in a teaching hospital and should represent the shortest times rather than the longest. This period spent immobile on a hard trolley dehydrated and in pain must account for many of the pressure sores observed in patients with a fractured neck of femur.

Pre-operative Admission to Ward

On first admission to the ward the patient is usually put on skin traction to stabilise the fracture, and given analgesia. The patient will however be held nil-by-mouth while waiting to go to the operating theatre. If the patient is not being adequately rehydrated by drip at this time, dehydration will continue to put the patient at risk of developing a pressure sore. In most units surgery for fractured neck of femur is done as an emergency. This does not necessarily mean that it is done quickly, merely that it is done outside working hours. The case queues with other 'emergency' cases such as Caesareans and abdominal emergencies, both of which for obvious reasons take priority over a fractured neck of femur. The result is that patients may wait nil-by-mouth on skin traction for long periods before surgery. From my own studies the median waiting time is around 12 hours from admission, the shortest period recorded being 2 hours and the longest 72 hours. During this waiting it may be difficult for the nursing staff to institute any regular turning schedule both because of the pain the patient is experiencing and because of the knowledge that the patient may be going down to the operating theatre at any time. They may spend a significant amount of this waiting time already on a 'canvas', so that it can happen that during this time the patient is not turned at all and is again at severe risk of developing a sore.

The Operation Room

Once anaesthetised, the patient is lifted onto the operating table. In the case of a displaced per-trochanteric fracture this involves transfer onto an orthopaedic table, a procedure which can only be performed by several people physically lifting the patient onto the table. As the patient is anaesthetised, there is the possibility of inexperienced or careless staff handling the patient in a cavalier manner. Once again skin damage can be the result.

The orthopaedic table itself is both hard and narrow to give good access to the surgeon (Figure 6.1). The buttocks are supported on a small, unpadded plate whose area varies according to the design. Some designs of sacral plate support the whole pelvis, others are so small that only a small area around the coccyx supports the whole weight of the lower body. Although this gives excellent access to the surgeon, it provides quite unacceptably high pressures to the sacral region. Even if carefully padded with wool, the area is far too small to reduce the local pressures to satisfactory levels, and the larger support should always be used. This should be carefully padded at least with wool and preferably with one of the purpose-built, weight-distributing foam pads. The central pole in the groin is used on this table to stabilise the patient on the narrow table and to provide a purchase for counter-traction when reducing the fracture. If the

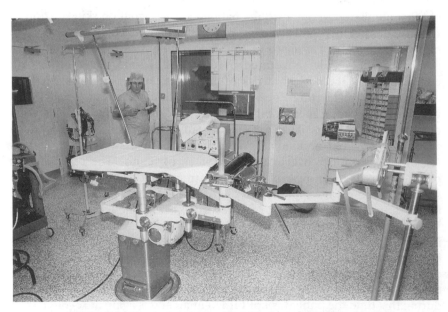

Figure 6.1   Typical orthopaedic table in an operating theatre

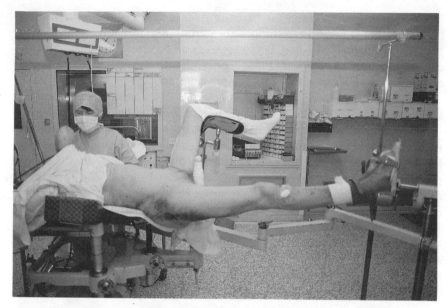

Figure 6.2 Common position of a patient during an operation

reduction traction is left on throughout the operation, the pole (even when padded) will produce a pressure sore deep in the groin over the adductors.

On the orthopaedic table the feet are supported in shoes attached to adjustable arms to allow positioning and traction to be applied to the legs (Figure 6.2). Poor positioning of the foot holder, inadequate padding, or traction left on throughout the operation can lead to the formation of heel sores or, more characteristically, sores over the achilles tendon where the counter of the shoe cuts into the heel.

Post-operatively, the aim is for the patient to get up and walk as soon as possible. Nevertheless, frail and elderly patients may spend some time in bed recovering from the surgery before mobilisation can be undertaken. During this time, if the heels are not protected then sores may appear in this area, while if the patient is not regularly turned both day and night sacral sores can also occur. These are made more likely if the patient is incontinent (as many are, either permanently or while recovering from the anaesthetic). Demented or confused patients may fret continuously in bed and rub heels or other parts of the body against the sheets. Their continuous movement may produce the very sores that movement normally prevents.

Because of the low level of care required for post-operative orthopaedic patients compared with some other surgical specialities, nursing levels on orthopaedic wards can fall to very low levels indeed. In some trauma orthopaedic wards it is not uncommon to have one trained and one student nurse covering more than 20 patients over a night shift. Under these circumstances it is well-nigh impossible for those staff to ensure that all patients are turned as often as is necessary to ensure that pressure sores cannot develop. Versluysen (1985) reports that in some units up to 40 per cent of the nurses' time is devoted to pressure area care.

It is often said (Jensen and Juncker, 1987) that elderly patients with a fractured neck of femur must be treated surgically because conservative treatment inevitably leads to pressure sores, hypostatic bronchopneumonia and urinary tract infections. This in turn leads to the death of the patient. In the author's experience this has not proved the case. In those few patients who were sound of mind and who refused surgery for a fractured neck of femur the long-term results were good. With adequate, trained nursing care it appears that there is no reason why a patient managed on a Thomas splint or on balanced traction should not heal without pressure sores or other complications. The resource implications of this type of management to the Health Service would be dire indeed and it is probable that this is the main reason why the conservative management of this common condition is currently held in such ill-favour.

Traction

It is not just in the management of fractured neck of femur that the association between conservative management and pressure sores is encouraging a move towards internal fixation of fractures with early mobilisation. In those fractures of the lower limb which cannot be held reduced by plaster of Paris, the safest and surest method of ensuring early union without infection or other complications is the use of traction. The advent of internal fixation, and in particular the locking intra-medullary nail, has led to a major change in the management of many fractures. This complex and demanding surgical treatment is attractive to surgeons for two reasons. The first is that it uses to the full the skills in which they are trained, and the second is that it allows early discharge of the patient so that the bed can be used for another patient. It is however not so clear that this is in the best interests of the patient. Without doubt he goes home earlier, but there is no evidence that the rate of union is better than with conservative management. There is however good evidence that the complications are not insignificant in terms of infection and other complications of surgery. The argument is however put forward that pressure sores are a complication of the conservative management of these young patients. The author's experience is that this is only the case in those units who routinely use internal fixation for the management of fractures and who therefore have little experience of setting up traction. The result is that the traction is not carefully monitored and pressure sores result. In units routinely using

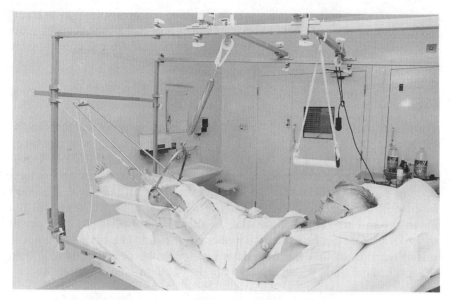

Figure 6.3 Patient with fracture managed by traction

traction these problems simply do not occur. The causes of pressure sores on traction (Figure 6.3) are very straightforward, and once understood by all staff should become a completely avoidable problem.

Imbalance

If balanced traction is being used the principle is that weights pulling in one direction to reduce the fracture must be balanced by an equal weight in the opposite direction. If not then the patient will move inexorably towards the unbalanced weight. The patient's efforts to hoist himself back up the bed merely allow the slide to be repeated as often as the patient has the will to return himself to the security of the centre of his bed. The continuous friction of his sacral area will inevitably lead to the formation of a pressure (friction) sore. Counter-traction to prevent this slipping is provided by tipping the bed so that the traction weights are effectively trying to draw the patient uphill. Once the tilt of the bed is correct the traction becomes 'balanced' and the patient effectively floats on his traction. The problem arises when the ward is cleaned or the patient is taken for an X-ray to check position. Traction beams make beds so tall that they will no longer pass through doorways or fit into a lift while they remain tilted for balanced traction. If the bed is placed flat for any reason then it must be put back onto the same tilt within minutes, otherwise the traction is no longer balanced and the patient will sooner or later develop a friction sore on the sacrum. Modern beds are easily taken off tilt by the press of a simple lever, so that any member of staff unaware of the importance of the tilt is capable of unbalancing the traction. If the trained ward staff are not continuously aware of this danger then pressure sores will result.

Heel Sores

These can occur on balanced traction if the traction is not set to hold the heels clear of the bed. If the weight of the patient's leg is being taken directly by the heel on the bed, friction sores can result. Rubber gloves filled with water can provide some protection but rely on the patient keeping perfectly still so that the heel does not slip off the glove. The very essence of balanced traction is that the patient should not keep still but move around to keep soft tissues healthy. Water-filled rubber gloves should therefore not be used with balanced traction. The best solution is to set up traction so that the heel does not touch the bed. If this fails then sheepskin heel pads which move with the foot provide a more effective solution.

REFERENCES

Duthie, R. B. (1981). In *Orthopaedic Services: Waiting times for Outpatient Appointments and In-patient Treatment*, DHSS, London, pp. 17–23

Ferris, B. (1983). Decubitus ulceration following prosthetic implantation for traumatic subcapital fractured neck of femur. A preventable condition? *Br. J. Clin. Pract.*, **37**(5), 175–177

Heyse-Moore, G. H., MacEachern, A. G. and Evans, D. C. J. (1983). Treatment of intertrochanteric fractures of the femur. A comparison of the Richards screw-plate and the Jewett nail-plate. *J. Bone Joint Surg.*, **65-B**, 262–267

Jensen, T. J. and Juncker, Y. (1987). Pressure sores common after hip operations. *Acta. Orthop. Scand.*, **58**, 209–211

Jordan, M. M. and Clark, M. O. (1977a). Report on the incidence of pressure sores in the patient community of the greater Glasgow Health Board Area on 21st January 1976. Bioengineering unit, University of Strathclyde, and the Greater Glasgow Health Board. Reported in Versluysen (1985)

Jordan, M. M., Nicol, S. M. and Melrose, A. L. (1977). Report on the incidence of pressure sores in the patient community of the Borders Health Board Area on 13th October 1976. Bioengineering unit, University of Strathclyde, and the Borders Health Board. Reported in Versluysen (1985)

Lienbach, I. S. and Barlow, F. A. (1973). 700 total hip replacements. Experience with six types. *Clin. Orthop.*, **95**, 174–192

Lowthian, P. (1979). Pressure sore prevalence. A survey of sores in orthopaedic patients. *Nursing Times*, **75**(9), 358–360

Sheppeard, H., Cleak, D. K., Ward, D. J. and O'Connor, B. T. (1980). A review of early mortality and morbidity in elderly patients following Charnley total hip replacement. *Arch. Orth. Traum. Surg.*, **97**, 243–248

Versluysen, M. (1985). Pressure sores in elderly patients. *J. Bone Joint Surg.*, **67-B**, 10–13

7

Geriatric Medicine

M. Bliss

INCIDENCE

About 9 per cent of patients in British hospitals today suffer from pressure sores (Barbenel *et al.*, 1977), but the incidence rises steeply with age, reaching 20 per cent in those over 70 years (Norton *et al.*, 1975, Jordan *et al.*, 1976). The highest incidence occurs in elderly patients with fractured neck of femur (66 per cent) (Versluysen, 1986). In orthopaedic and geriatric wards, 30–50 per cent of patients are likely either to have pressure sores or to require special management to prevent them (Hibbs, 1982). The prevalence of sores in the community is generally lower than in hospital, but is similar in patients with similar degrees of disability (Jordan, 1979).

AETIOLOGY

Predisposing Diseases

The liability of older patients to develop pressure sores appears to be related mainly to the increase in neurological and cardiovascular disease with age (Jordan, 1979; Versluysen, 1986). Neurological disease, including Alzheimer's, Parkinson's, cerebrovascular disease and the 'psychoses', may alter the appreciation of pressure pain, reduce mobility, or affect autonomic responses to ischaemia (Guttmann, 1976). Cardiovascular disease affects local blood flow, especially peripheral vascular disease, which is the chief cause of the high incidence of sores of the heel in elderly compared with young patients (four times commoner in smokers than in non-smokers (Barton and Barton, 1978)). Foot sores also occur frequently in patients with neuro-arteriopathy due to diabetes mellitus and rheumatoid arthritis (Jordan *et al.*, 1977). Elderly patients who do not have neurological or vascular disease are probably no more susceptible to pressure sores than young patients. However, any patient of any age who is sufficiently ill may develop pressure ischaemia.

65

Illness

The precipitating cause of pressure necrosis is almost invariably illness or other form of stress (Roaf, 1976; Barton and Barton, 1978). Healthy old people, including those with greatly reduced mobility, do not normally develop pressure sores, but the same patients may become acutely vulnerable following the onset of an intercurrent illness, or trauma, at home or in hospital. Fewer pressure sores occur in the community, because fewer very sick patients are nursed at home – the onset of pressure necrosis itself frequently being the cause of admission to hospital. Fifteen per cent of all sores are present on admission, and of the remainder, 70 per cent develop during the following 2 weeks when patients are most ill (Norton *et al.*, 1975; Versluysen, 1986). Sores which occur later are usually associated with complications of the original illness, or with new intercurrent illness, or with progressive deterioration eventually leading to death.

Nursing Management

Although the poor general condition of the patient is the chief cause of the high incidence of sores following admission to hospital, medical and nursing management are also very important. Versluysen (1986) has shown that newly admitted, acutely ill or injured patients may be left lying on hard trolleys in casualty and X-ray departments without pressure relief for up to 6 hours, and similar periods may later be spent awaiting transfer to theatre, or on unprotected operating tables (see also Chapter 6). Sores may be caused by casts or traction apparatus, or simply by hard hospital beds, rough sheets and drawsheets (Lowthian, 1983). The practice of nursing susceptible patients in chairs to prevent pressure sores is also likely to do more harm than good (Lowthian, 1977). In a comprehensive survey of pressure sores, Barbenel *et al.* (1977) found more sores, including more necrotic sores, in patients being nursed in chairs than in bed. Low staffing levels are often cited as the cause of the high incidence of sores in geriatric wards, but the acute susceptibility of the patients and inappropriate methods of care are likely to be at least as important.

PATHOLOGY

Sores occur mainly over bony prominences, e.g. over the sacrum (33 per cent), heels (18 per cent), ischial tuberosities (18 per cent) and greater trochanters (11 per cent) (Jordan, 1979), but they may occur in any situation where there has been excessive pressure, e.g. on the shoulders or elbows, or under a bandage (Figure 7.1). In an elderly patient, any

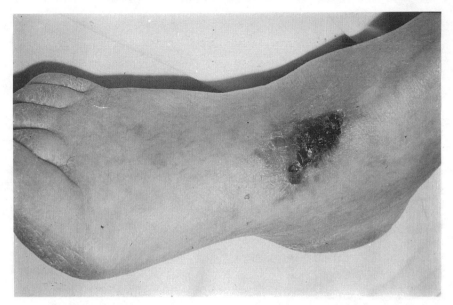

Figure 7.1   Pressure sore caused by a bandage

localised area of discoloration or ulceration should be assumed to be due to pressure and a search made for a possible source before considering other causes.

Eighty per cent of sores in elderly patients are superficial, involving only the epidermis and dermis, and 20 per cent are deep (Norton *et al.*, 1975). Superficial sores occur mainly in weak, immobile, incontinent patients who are confined to bed or chairs, but who are not acutely ill. They are often associated with urine rashes, and appear to be due to a combination of pressure and friction of macerated skin. Deep or full thickness sores only occur in very sick patients. They may be superimposed on the site of a superficial sore, but more often they appear suddenly in an area of previously normal skin, about 8 to 24 hours following the period of pressure (Barton and Barton, 1978). The dead tissue presents initially as a red or blackish patch, or a localised area of swelling on the skin. This demarcates to form a black eschar with surrounding oedema and hyper-aemia (Figure 7.2). Over the next 2–4 weeks, the dead cells liquefy and break down to discharge quantities of foul-smelling fluid, and slough, leaving an empty cavity. The shape of the sore depends on the area of original damage caused by the pressure. This is usually greater in the deep tissues than in the skin, so that a typical sore has overhanging edges and often deep sinuses which may extend for many centimetres. Over the ensuing month, the wound contracts to about half its original size and most of the sinuses close. The remaining defect then slowly fibroses to form a

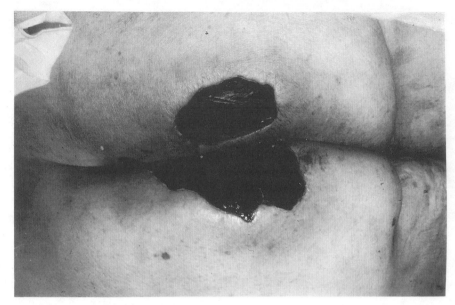

Figure 7.2   Necrotic pressure sore of the buttocks

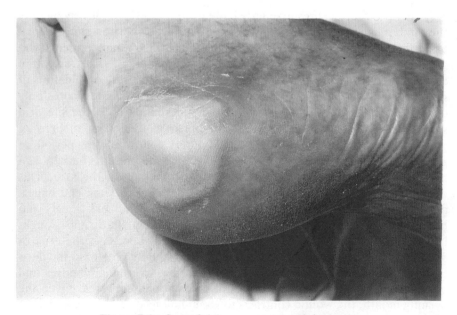

Figure 7.3   Superficial pressure sore of the heel

depressed scar. As soon as it breaks down, the sore invariably becomes infected with pathogenic bacteria, but these do not appear to retard healing. The local inflammation and accompanying pyrexia and leucocytosis are reactions to the presence of dead tissue, not infection, and subside spontaneously once natural debridement begins.

Depending on whether they are superficial or deep, sores of the heel present as colourless or reddish-black blisters (Figure 7.3). Necrotic heel sores develop very adherent black eschars which separate much more slowly than those of trunk sores.

PROGNOSIS

Fifty per cent of all elderly patients who develop pressure sores die within 4 months, including 90 per cent of those with necrotic sores of the trunk. Full-thickness heel sores have a better prognosis, but are often difficult to heal because of their poor blood supply.

PREVENTION

Identifying Susceptible Patients – the Pressure Sore Prediction Score

The chief difficulty in preventing pressure sores lies in deciding which patients need prophylaxis before sores appear. Norton *et al.* (1975) devised the 'pressure sore prediction score' (Table 7.1). This has been widely used in research and practice, but has two major disadvantages: it needs to be assessed daily, which is usually impossible with large numbers of patients, and progressive deterioration of the score is more likely to be significant than the actual level. Thus a very disabled, incontinent patient may have a chronically low Norton score in the danger zone below 14, and yet remain free of sores, because his general physical condition is 'good', but subsequent *reduction of the total* caused by deterioration of his health

Table 7.1 The Norton pressure sore prediction score

	Physical condition	Mental state	Activity	Mobility	Incontinence
4	good	alert	ambulant	full	continent
3	fair	confused	with help	limited	occasionally
2	poor	apathetic	chairfast	very limited	usually urine
1	bad	stuporose	in bed	immobile	doubly

A score of 14 or below indicates susceptibility to sores

to 'fair' or 'poor', due, for example, to the onset of a urinary tract infection, is highly likely to be followed by a pressure sore. The inference is that a score is probably unnecessary, and that it may be easier and safer simply to identify certain susceptible groups of patients, i.e. *patients aged over 70 years*, and those with *neurological disease* and *paraplegia*, for whom pressure prophylaxis should automatically be considered whenever and wherever they become ill. Suitable regimes and equipment can then be kept in readiness for immediate use.

All patients aged over 70 years being admitted to hospital should be considered as being likely to need pressure care for at least the first week of stay. This should include those being admitted for holiday relief, as requests for relief admissions are often precipitated by a deterioration in the patient's health and therefore dependency. The stress of transfer to hospital itself may also be sufficient to cause susceptibility to pressure sores. Similarly, all elderly in-patients in hospitals or nursing homes, or residents in old people's homes or in the community, should be started on a programme of pressure care from the moment they develop any new illness or trauma. Physical signs in old people are often non-specific, so that symptoms such as confusion or aggression, dehydration, loss of appetite, or the onset of incontinence or constipation, should be regarded as being due to illness. Patients who require sedative drugs for an acute confusional state are doubly at risk, both from the illness causing the confusion, and from the sedative and Parkinsonian side effects of the drug. Butyrophenone preparations are especially liable to precipitate massive necrosis. Patients who develop drowsiness on these drugs should be put to bed and given full pressure prophylaxis. Finally, any evidence of pressure damage itself, for example, unfading red patches on the heels, is an extremely important, non-specific sign of illness in an elderly person, indicating the need both for urgent medical investigation and immediate pressure relief.

Programme of Pressure Care

The principles of emergency pressure relief for an old person are as follows:

- Nurse the patient mainly or wholly in bed, lying as flat as possible.
- Provide a heel fleece, covering the whole of the lower third of the bed.
- Provide an end-of-bed cradle.
- Provide a pressure-relieving mattress and/or carry out regular repositioning.

All acutely ill, elderly patients who are susceptible to pressure sores should be nursed mainly in bed. Patients recover from illness more quickly if they are nursed in bed and pressure can be more easily relieved if their weight is widely distributed lying down than when they are sitting in chairs. There is no reliable evidence that nursing old people in chairs improves chest disease or prevents venous thrombosis, and it is likely to exacerbate cardiac and renal insufficiency and increase oedema (Guite *et al.*, 1988). The risk of bedrest causing calcium loss and contractures is far less important than the need to prevent sores, which themselves may greatly prolong the debilitated state and its attendant complications.

The bed should be provided with an end-of-bed cradle to lift the weight of the blankets off the feet. The whole of the lower third should be covered by a nursing fleece with anchoring flaps at the sides and extending up under the draw sheet to prevent patients getting their feet underneath it. A fleece is a valuable aid for preventing sores of the feet in patients with peripheral vascular disease, and is more comfortable and effective than heel pads or 'gutters' strapped onto the legs.

The best-known method for preventing pelvic sores is 'two-hourly turning'. This was originally developed in spinal injury units, but it is less satisfactory for geriatric patients. Old people frequently need to be nursed sitting up in bed for cardiac or chest disease, or have poor balance and dislike lying on their sides. They may scream when they are moved, upsetting other patients, or move out of position. Simple 'side-to-side' turning on an ordinary bed is also liable to cause severe sores over the hips. Turning regimes in spinal patients are carefully regulated to minimise the time spent on these vulnerable areas (Lowthian, 1985), and the bed surface is modified by pillows (Guttmann, 1976) or special mattresses (Scales, 1982) to relieve pressure under bony prominences. Whenever possible, however, elderly patients much prefer to be nursed on pressure-relieving mattresses on which they do not require frequent repositioning.

Pressure-relieving Mattresses

There are three basic kinds of pressure-relieving mattress: turning beds and frames, low-pressure and flotation beds, and alternating pressure beds. Turning beds (Lowthian, 1977) are alarming and unsuitable for geriatric patients. Low-pressure 'soft' beds, such as especially structured foam (e.g. Vaperm–Scales, 1982) or slit foam (e.g. Polyflote–Reswick and Rogers, 1976) mattresses, silicore mattresses (e.g. Spenco–Stapleton, 1986) and non-flotation water beds (e.g. Western Medical–Lowthian, 1977) are more acceptable, but tension in the surface membrane, similar to that which occurs in a hammock (e.g. Egerton net bed–Lowthian, 1977), may produce shear stresses and tissue distortion over bony prominences, sufficient to cause sores unless the patients are also repositioned regularly.

Static air mattresses have been designed which reduce shearing forces (e.g. Roho–Graebe, 1981), but all static air mattresses lose air with the risk of bottoming unless they are regularly checked and reinflated. The Simpson Edinburgh bed (Torrance, 1981) is inflated mechanically, but does not prevent sores without regular turning of the patient. The Mediscus low-air-loss bed (Scales, 1982; Krouskop *et al.*, 1984) provides a low-pressure surface on which patients can be nursed mainly in one position, but requires manual adjustment, and is non-portable and expensive.

Flotation beds, such as the Beaufort Winchester water bed (Neumark, 1981) and the Clinitron air fluidised bead bed (Krouskop *et al.*, 1984), are able to prevent sores without additional repositioning of the patient, but are disliked by most old people because they reduce their ability to help themselves. Getting patients in and out of bed, feeding, dressing and toiletting are also very difficult on a flotation water bed, and many orthopaedic procedures and cardiac massage are impossible. The Clinitron has been designed to overcome some of these problems by enabling the flotation action to be switched off when required, but it is bulky, difficult to install and prohibitively expensive (hire charge of upward of £385 per week).

Alternating-pressure air mattresses (APAMs) are potentially the most acceptable, convenient and reasonably priced aids for elderly patients. They consist of two or more alternating series of air cells which inflate and deflate every 5–10 minutes under the patient, thus constantly altering the supporting points of pressure on the body. Providing the cells are large enough (about 10 cm), to raise bony prominences such as the sacrum and hips clear of the underlying surface of the bed, and providing the systems are sufficiently robust and well serviced not to break down in use, they provide good pressure protection (Wright, 1980). The most widely used APAMs in Britain today are the Pegasus airwave bed (Exton-Smith *et al.*, 1982) (Figure 7.4), the large-celled Ripple bed (Bliss *et al.*, 1967) and bubble pads. The Pegasus bed has a double bank of cells which permits relief of pressure under even very heavy or emaciated patients. It prevents and heals necrotic sores in patients being nursed in one position, but the active movement may occasionally aggravate friction sores. It should always be used with a double underblanket or a nursing fleece. It is suitable for orthopaedic patients and can be instantly deflated to permit cardiac massage, if necessary. The large-celled Ripple bed can also provide good relief of pressure in patients being nursed in one position, but present models are mechanically unreliable (Bliss, 1979). The small-celled Ripple bed (cells 5 cm in diameter) and bubble pads do not have enough depth to prevent pressure sores without repositioning in most patients. Ripple beds and bubble pads are easily portable by one person, so that they are useful in an emergency, and in the community. The Pegasus bed is more cumbersome but can still be installed fairly easily on most hospital or

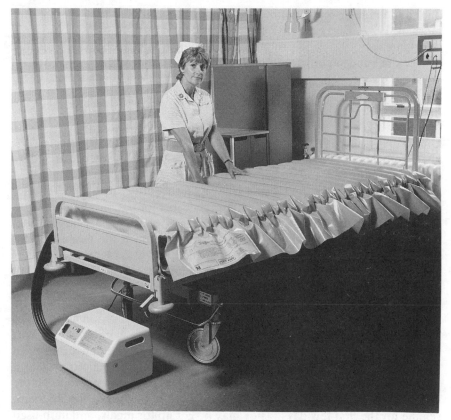

Figure 7.4 Pegasus airwave bed

domestic beds. APAMs are usually unnoticed by sick elderly patients, and cause minimal disturbance to nursing.

Whatever type of pressure-relieving mattress is used, the bed linen should be of fine material and only lightly tucked in. Thick draw macs, draw sheets and incontinence pads are especially damaging on soft mattresses. Night wear should also be of fine, soft material and generously cut. Immobile or contracted patients should have a pillow placed between the knees to prevent pressure on the legs or genitals.

Skin Care

The skin should be kept as clean and dry as possible by regular changing of incontinent patients, or catheterisation, but it is unlikely that specific local treatments which are often recommended have any benefit other than that due to the regular repositioning required for their application (Fernie and Dornan, 1976). Barrier sprays and creams do not prevent pressure necrosis (Norton *et al.*, 1975) and probably afford only minimal protection against urine rashes and superficial sores.

Progressive Programme of Pressure Care

Unless the patient is to be admitted to hospital immediately, pressure care needs to begin at home. Heel fleeces and APAMs can easily be carried by general practitioners and district nurses in their cars, and a tray or a pillow in the bottom of the bed can serve as a substitute for a bed-cradle. Two-hourly repositioning is usually impracticable for patients being nursed at home, so that every effort should be made to provide a large-celled Ripple or bubble pad, preferably on the day on which the patient is first seen. This may be replaced by a more dependable system such as a Pegasus mattress later if domiciliary care is to be continued.

In the accident and emergency department, trolleys being used for old people should be protected with soft mattresses. Patients should be admitted to the wards for more intensive pressure care as soon as possible. Those needing to go to theatre should have schedules worked out so that, as soon as practicable, they may be given drinks to relieve dehydration. In theatre, the operating table must be protected by a soft mattress and a pillow should be placed under the patient's calves to relieve pressure on the heels. Post-operatively, all patients should be nursed on a low-pressure regime for the first few days. They may be got up for meals, and mobilised gently as soon as their condition permits, but should be returned to rest on their beds for the greater part of each day. This regime should be continued until their general condition and mobility show that they are no longer in danger of pressure ischaemia. The pressure-relieving mattress can then be removed in order to facilitate rehabilitation, but should be replaced immediately if there is any subsequent deterioration in the patient's general condition or pressure areas.

Support Cushions

As has already been discussed, acutely ill, elderly patients who are liable to pressure sores are best nursed mainly in bed. They should not be got up for more than 2–4 hours daily, during which time a comfortable chair with a fleece is usually adequate protection. Support cushions (e.g. gel–Spence, 1967; Jay Flolite–Swain, 1987; Roho air–Graebe, 1981) are therefore only indicated for fit old people confined to wheelchairs. Even then, it must be remembered that old people do not have the same strength as young patients to do 'push-ups' (Barbenel, 1984), so that they are likely to need a siesta to provide a radical change of position at least once during the day.

HEALING PRESSURE SORES

Nutrition

In elderly patients, nutritional support, e.g. with protein, vitamin C (Husain, 1953) or zinc (Hallbrook and Lammer, 1972) supplements, is much less important for healing sores than relief of pressure. Sores in old people are never sufficiently protracted to cause the chronic, septic states and amyloidosis seen in young patients (Tribe and Silver, 1969). In elderly patients, the appetite usually responds well to simple measures such as bed rest, adequate pain and pressure relief, and frequent drinks.

Persistent refusal of fluid and food are often due to oral thrush or faecal impaction, both of which are extremely common in patients with pressure sores. The mouth and rectum must always be examined and vigorous, repeated treatment given if necessary. Patients who continue to have a poor appetite are likely to be dying. They may be offered protein drinks, but enteral feeding is seldom appropriate or of lasting benefit.

Pain Relief

Unlike pressure sores in young patients, who often have anaesthesia due to neurological disease, both superficial and deep sores in old people are usually extremely painful. Effective analgesia is essential. Anti-inflammatory drugs are useless and merely likely to cause side effects and to retard healing (Barton and Barton, 1978). For small superficial sores, careful positioning on a nursing fleece or a pressure-relieving mattress is usually sufficient, but patients with extensive superficial or necrotic sores are likely to require diamorphine. Five milligrams are usually adequate, but larger doses should be used if necessary. The drug is best given orally as an elixir 4-hourly for at least the first week until the sloughs have begun to separate. Anti-emetics are seldom necessary, but additional laxatives are almost always required. Addiction never occurs, and the drug can be tailed off as soon as healing is established. Most patients become more relaxed and alert, and begin to eat and drink and to move more freely as soon as their pain is relieved. Those who do not are usually dying but still likely to benefit from adequate analgesia.

Pressure Care

Trunk sores usually heal readily once pressure is relieved. All weight should be removed from the area if possible, but healing will still take place on a Pegasus APAM or a flotation bed if a patient with multiple sores has to lie on the site of a sore. The mattress should be chosen to suit individual needs. Some patients with extensive sores find the Pegasus bed uncomfortable, but this may be helped by adequate analgesia. Superficial sores need to be exposed by careful positioning to ensure optimum healing. The Mediscus bed is usually well tolerated, but it requires manual supervision and is expensive, and sores in patients being nursed on it should be exposed wherever possible. Dressings may be difficult on a flotation water bed. The Clinitron is effective, but is rarely justified when other, much cheaper mattresses are available.

Patients with trunk sores should not be allowed to sit out of bed for more than 1–2 hours each day. They may be dressed and got up for meals and physiotherapy, and even encouraged to walk if practicable, but should return to rest on their beds at all other times.

Patients with heel sores should also be put to bed on a pressure-relieving mattress. This prevents the development of trunk sores and relieves oedema, which is almost invariably present in patients with foot sores. Oedema retards healing by reducing the circulation (Wright, 1980) in tissues which are usually already jeopardised by a poor arterial blood supply. Attempts to elevate the legs to the level of the pelvis while sitting in a chair cause intolerable discomfort and are merely liable to increase pressure on both the heels and the sacral area. Diuretics alone are ineffective for relieving leg oedema in these patients. Elastic stockings are also ineffective, and risk causing further pressure damage to the skin (Figure 7.1). The patient should rest on his bed with his heels suspended over a pillow or foam wedge. If he is reasonably well, he may be dressed and encouraged to walk as much as possible. Once the fluid overload has been relieved and the local inflammation has subsided (usually in about one week), he may be allowed to sit in a chair, with his feet on the floor, for gradually increasing periods each day.

Local Treatment

Local treatment should be kept to a minimum. Sloughs of trunk sores seldom need medical or surgical debridement, as they separate naturally within about 3 weeks once pressure has been relieved from the area. Surgery merely exposes the patient to the hazards of an operation and may increase the risk of disseminating infection. In patients treated conservatively, routine 'swabbing' and treatment with antibiotics is unnecessary.

Side effects from systemic antibiotics are common in elderly patients, and local antibiotics are liable to cause skin sensitisation. Antiseptics such as 'Eusol', hydrogen peroxide and povidone iodine should also be avoided whenever possible, as they damage granulation tissue (Brennan and Leaper, 1985) and may even prevent eventual healing (Barnett, 1987). In elderly patients, pressure sores do not need to be packed as the sinuses virtually never seal and form abscesses. Packing merely increases local pressure on the walls of the cavity, delays natural debridement and wound contraction, and greatly increases pain. Silastic foam is probably less damaging than gauze (Wood *et al.*, 1977), but it is not known if this, or packing with granules such as dextronomer beads (Masser, 1983), has any advantage over no packing. Even very large pressure sores which are left empty heal rapidly once they are relieved of pressure. They should simply be syringed daily with normal saline and dressed with sheets of gauze strapped across the opening. If required, honey placed in the wound appears to reduce bacterial colonisation and odour (Cavanagh *et al.*, 1970), and may possibly accelerate healing (Anonymus, 1988).

Superficial sores in the sacral area are often more difficult to treat than deep sores. All types of dressing, including occlusive dressings such as Opsite (Chrisp, 1977) or Granuflex (Mertz *et al.*, 1985), tend to rumple and cause further skin damage in this weight-bearing area. Every effort must be made to remove all pressure from the site. Where this is impossible it is often best to leave the wound exposed and to sit the patient directly on a nursing fleece.

Unlike trunk sores, healing of full-thickness sores of the heel may be hastened by debridement of the very tenacious sloughs by a proteolytic cream (e.g. Varidase–Poulson *et al.*, 1983) under an occlusive dressing. The debriding agent should be discontinued as soon as all the necrotic tissue has separated and the wound dressed simply with unmedicated paraffin gauze.

Surgery

Pressure sores in elderly patients seldom require surgery. Even large sores of the trunk usually heal readily with relief of pressure and avoidance of unsuitable local treatment. Those which are less responsive usually occur in very deteriorated patients for whom protracted nursing on a pressure-relieving bed is likely to be necessary in order to prevent further ischaemia, and in whom the presence of a granulating sore is probably less hazardous than surgical attempts at closure. However, operative treatment can be extremely helpful in a healthy patient whose rehabilitation is being delayed by a large trunk sore. Complete healing can be achieved in about two weeks with radical excision and closure of the wound by rotation skin flaps

(Keller and Shaw, 1985). Split skin grafting may also occasionally help to heal refractory sores of the feet.

REFERENCES

Anonymus (1988). Honey provides sweet cure for wounds. *New Scientist*, 119, 1620, 36

Barbenel, J. C. (1984). Movements of paraplegic patients in wheelchairs. *Care, Science and Practice*, **3**, 2, 60–64

Barbenel, J. C., Jordan, M. M., Nicol, S. M. and Clark, M. O. (1977). Incidence of pressure sores in the Greater Glasgow Health Board Area. *Lancet*, **2**, 548–550

Barnett, S. E. (1987). Histology of the human pressure sore. *Care, Science and Practice*, **5**, 2, 13–18

Barton, A. A. (1970). The pathogenesis and inhibition of pressure sores. MD Thesis, University of London

Barton, A. and Barton, M. (1978). The management and prevention of pressure sores. Faber, London and Boston

Bliss, M. R. (1979). The use of Ripple beds in hospitals. *Hospital and Health Services Review*, **74**, 190–193

Bliss, M. R., McLaren, R. and Exton-Smith, A. N. (1967). Preventing pressure sores in hospital: controlled trial of a large celled Ripple mattress. *British Medical Journal*, **1**, 394–397

Brennan, S. S. and Leaper, D. J. (1985). The effect of antiseptics on the healing wound: a study using the rabbit ear chamber. *British Journal of Surgery*, **72**, 780–782

Cavanagh, D., Beazley, J. and Ostapowicze, F. (1970). Radical operation for carcinoma of the vulva – a new approach to wound healing. *The Journal of Obstetrics and Gynaecology of the British Commonwealth*, **77**, 1037–1040

Chrisp, M. (1977). New treatment for pressure sores. *Nursing Times*, **73**, 1203–1205

Exton-Smith, A. N., Overstall, P. W., Wedgewood, J. and Wallace, G. (1982). Use of the 'Airwave system' to prevent pressure sores in hospital. *Lancet*, **1**, 1288–1290

Fernie, G. R. and Dornan, J. (1976). The problem of clinical trials with new systems of preventing or healing decubiti. In Kenedi, R. M., Cowden, J. M. and Scales, J. T. (eds), *Bedsore Biomechanics*, Macmillan Press, London and Basingstoke, pp. 315–320

Graebe, R. H. (1981). Static forces – cushion. *Care, Science and Practice*, **1**, 1, 50–53

Guite, H. F., Bliss, M. R., Mainwaring-Burton, R. W., Thomas, J. M. and Drury, P. L. (1988). Hypothesis: posture is one of the determinents of the circadian rhythm of urine flow and electrolyte excretion in elderly female patients. *Age and Ageing*, **17**, 241–248

Guttmann, L. (1976). The prevention and treatment of pressure sores. In Kenedi, R. M., Cowden, J. M. and Scales, J. T. (eds), *Bedsore Biomechanics*, Macmillan Press, London and Basingstoke, pp. 153–159

Hallbrook, T. and Lammer, E. (1972). Serum zinc and healing of venous leg ulcers. *Lancet*, **2**, 780–782

Hibbs, P. (1982). Pressure sores: a system of prevention. *Nursing Mirror*, **155**, 5, 25–29

Husain, T. (1953). An experimental study of some pressure effects on tissues with reference to the bedsore problem. *Journal of Pathology and Bacteriology*, **66**, 347–354

Jordan, M. M. (1979). Report on pressure sores in the elderly. Further information from the survey of the patient community of the Greater Glasgow Health Board Area on 21st January 1976. Bioengineering Unit, University of Strathclyde

Jordan, M. M., Nicol, S. M. and Melrose, A. L. (1977). Report on the incidence of pressure sores in the patient community of the Borders Health Board Area on 13th October 1976. Bioengineering Unit, University of Strathclyde, and the Borders Health Board

Keller, A. and Shaw, W. (1985). Technique in the surgery of pressure sores. In Lee, B. Y. (ed.), *Chronic Ulcers of the Skin*, McGraw-Hill, New York, pp. 171–185

Krouskop, T., Williams, R. and Krebs, M. (1984). The effectiveness of air flotation beds. *Care, Science and Practice*, **4**, 2, 9–11

Lowthian, P. (1977). A review of pressure sore prophylaxis. *Nursing Mirror*, Suppl., 17 March, vii–xv

Lowthian, P. (1983). Nursing aspects of pressure sore prevention. In Barbenel, J. C., Forbes, C. D. and Lowe, G. D. O. (eds), *Pressure Sores*, Macmillan Press, London and Basingstoke

Lowthian, P. (1985). Preventing pressure sores. *Nursing Mirror*, **160**, 25, 18–20

Masser, M. R. (1983). An objective comparison of Debrisan with cotton gauze. *Care, Science and Practice*, **2**, 4, 27–33

Mertz, P. M., Marshall, D. A. and Eaglestern, W. H. (1985). Occlusive wound dressings to prevent bacterial invasion and wound infection. *Journal of the American Academy of Dermatology*, **12**, 4, 662–668

Neumark, O. W. (1981). Deformation, not pressure, is the prime cause of pressure sores. *Care, Science and Practice*, **1**, 1, 41–43

Norton, D., McLaren, R. and Exton-Smith, A. N. (1975). *An Investigation of Geriatric Nursing Problems in Hospital*, Churchill-Livingstone, Edinburgh

Poulsen, J., Kristensen, U. N., Brygger, H. E. and Delikaris, P. (1983). Treatment of infected surgical wounds with Varidase. *Acta Chirurgica Scandinavia*, **149**, 3, 245–248

Reswick, J. B. and Rogers, J. (1976). Experience at Ranchos Los Amigos Hospital with devices and techniques to prevent pressure sores. In Kenedi, R. M., Cowden, J. M. and Scales, J. T. (eds), *Bedsore Biomechanics*, Macmillan Press, London and Basingstoke, pp. 301–310

Roaf, R. (1976). The causation and prevention of bedsores. In Kenedi, R. M., Cowden, J. M. and Scales, J. T. (eds), *Bedsore Biomechanics*, Macmillan Press, London and Basingstoke, pp. 5–9

Scales, J. T. (1982). Pressure sore prevention. *Care, Science and Practice*, **1**, 2, 9–17

Spence, W. (1967). Gel support for the prevention of decubitus ulcers. *Archives of Physical Medicine and Rehabilitation*, **28**, 283–288

Stapleton, M. (1986). Preventing pressure – an evaluation of three products. *British Journal of Geriatric Nursing*, **6**, 2, 23–25

Swain, I. (1987). Objective evaluation of patient support surfaces. Paper read at the autumn conference of the Tissue Viability Society at the University of Surrey, Guildford

Torrance, C. (1981). Pressure sores – mechanical devices. *Nursing Times*, **77**, 16, 13–16

Tribe, C. and Silver, J. R. (1969). *Renal Failure in Paraplegia*. Pitman, London

Versluysen, M. (1986). How elderly patients with femoral neck fracture develop pressure sores in hospital. *British Medical Journal*, **292**, 1311–1313

Wood, R. A. B., Williams, R. H. P. and Hughes, L. E. (1977). Foam elastomer dressing in the management of open granulating wounds: experience with 250 patients. *British Journal of Surgery*, **64**, 554–557

Wright, W. B. (1980). Pressure sores. Sensible precautions which aid prevention. *Geriatric Medicine*, **10**, 2, 9

8

The Severely Disabled

George Cochrane

DEFINITION

The cells of the body die if the flow of blood in the capillary bed is insufficient to bring oxygen, carbohydrates and amino acids for their metabolic needs and remove carbon dioxide and the products of catabolism, and maintain physical and chemical balance within narrow limits. A pressure sore is ischaemic necrosis of tissue which has been subjected to prolonged pressure against an external surface such as a bed, splint or wheelchair. Tissues overlying a bony prominence of sacrum, ischial tuberosities, greater trochanters, lateral malleoli and heels are especially susceptible. Not only superficial tissues but also muscle and bone can be affected.

The Stages of Formation of a Trophic Ulcer

There are four stages corresponding to tissue layers and extent of necrosis. The first, which is the most difficult to record, consists of skin discoloration which may be persisting redness, blood under the skin, oedema and induration and epidermal blistering; in the second there is an epithelial defect, a superficial pressure sore with a break in the skin at least 5 mm in diameter; in the third there is destruction of the epidermis and dermis but without a cavity; and in the fourth there is a subcutaneous cavity with necrosis extending to muscle and perhaps to bone with periostitis progressing to osteomyelitis with a possibility of septic arthritis, pathological fracture, septicaemia and death. Necrosis does not always begin superficially but may start in muscle overlying bone.

DISEASES AND DISORDERS IN WHICH RISKS ARE HIGH

The dangers of trophic ulcers are foremost in acute and chronic diseases of the very old, and in severe advanced disorders much earlier in life in multiple sclerosis, diseases of the spinal cord, spina bifida (particularly if associated with hydrocephalus), severe cerebral palsy, stroke, advanced rheumatoid arthritis and diabetes mellitus. In the presence of these diseases, vigilance must be intense and resolute.

Multiple Sclerosis

This is progressive, unpredictable and variable and caused by patches of inflammation and loss of neural myelin sheath in any part of the brain and spinal cord, bringing about mental, motor, sensory and autonomic disorders. Myelin is a complex of lipoprotein ensheathing nerve fibres and promoting the transmission of nerve impulses along the axon. The disease affects women more than men and the median survival time is more than 35 years. Bilateral corticospinal tract involvement is common with increased tone, spasticity and weakened movements. The balanced actions of agonist and antagonist muscles are lost. Fibrosis in the shortened muscles and around joints leads to contractures and these fixed deformities impose abnormal postures. Cerebellar lesions cause movements to be irregular, tremulous and ineffective, and the combination of spasticity and cerebellar ataxia may be totally disabling. Loss of sensations of pain and position are frequent. In severe disease, bladder and rectal incontinence and urinary tract infection are common. Apathy, lack of judgement and reactive depression are also usual, and late in the disease all the culprits of trophic ulcers are gathering. Invalidism may be prevented or postponed by physiotherapy, correct positioning in bed and in sitting, prompt treatment of infections, condom drainage of urine in men and intermittent catheterisation or indwelling suprapubic catheterisation in women. Baclofen, at daily doses of 30–90 mg, reduces spasticity by inhibiting the spinal cord reflexes and may facilitate active and passive movements.

Mechanical Compression of the Spinal Cord

Development of this disorder may be acute, sub-acute or chronic. Acute compression is usually by injury, sub-acute by neoplasm, epidural abscess or haematoma, and chronic by a bony or cartilagenous protrusion into the spinal canal or a slowly growing extra-medullary tumour. Compression of the cord leads to motor weakness at and below the segmental level of the compression in a paraplegic pattern. The site and extent of the lesion determine whether sensory and sphincter deficits occur. The optimum treatment is surgical decompression and removal of the cause, and, in the case of epidural abscess, eradication of identified infection.

Syringomyelia

This is a fluid-filled cavity within the substance of the spinal cord. About half the lesions are congenital, occurring in the cervical area and often presenting in adolescence or early adult life, and half occur in association with intra-medullary tumors. The expanding cavity disrupts spinothalamic neurones, causing impairment of appreciation of pain, warmth and cold on the contralateral side of the body, and interrupts the lateral columns, causing spasticity and weakness in the trunk and legs. Trophic lesions through loss of protective sensation lead to painless burns and ulcers on the hands, sometimes painless disorganised joints in the upper limbs, and pressure sores. *Acute transverse myelitis* affects both grey and white matter in one or more adjacent thoracic segments of the spinal cord and may be caused by viral infections, vasculitis or intravenous use of heroin or amphetamine, but usually the cause is not found. Below the lesion there is partial or complete motor and sensory loss and loss of control of the bladder and bowel.

Dysplastic Congenital Conditions of the Spine (Including Spina Bifida)

In these, the sac protruding through the defective closure of the spinal column may contain meninges and spinal cord and nerve roots. The spinal defect is commonest in the lumbar and next the lower thoracic and sacral regions, and may extend over three to six vertebral segments. Closure of the defect soon after birth assures at least a temporary survival and thorough examination of the child and counselling of the parents should precede intervention. In 80 per cent of cases hydrocephalus will develop and insertion of a cerebrospinal fluid shunt is required. The prognosis is determined by the number and severity of abnormalities and associated congenital defects and is worst for those with complete paralysis, hydrocephalus, kyphosis and early hydronephrosis. In hydrocephalus, verbal abilities exceed skills in performance and self-neglect of the paralysed and insensitive part of the body is usual. Years of insistent training through childhood and adolescence in inspecting, washing and drying the skin, taking care in transfers and in the choice of seats and clothing, frequently relieving pressure on the buttocks and completely avoiding pressure if there is erythema, oedema or subcutaneous induration is often unrewarded.

Cerebral Palsy

A non-progressive motor disorder resulting from gestational or perinatal damage to the central nervous system, this is characterised by impairment of voluntary movement. Of the four main categories, namely spastic, athetoid, ataxic and mixed, spastic is the most common, representing about 70 per cent of cases. Diplegia connotes the dominant involvement of the legs. The affected limbs are usually under-developed, the muscles are hypertonic, and if there is severe spasticity inequality in the tone and power of contraction of the muscles of the trunk and limbs leads to scoliosis, obliquity of the pelvis and contractures with the legs displaced to one side. Spastic quadriplegia is often associated with disabling mental retardation, corticobulbar impairment of oral, lingual and palatal movements causes dysarthria, and there may be severe urinary and faecal incontinence. Inability to stand and walk leads to confinement to bed and chair. Spasticity of the extensor muscles of the trunk and lower limbs tends to apply the load in sitting not on the buttocks but on the sacrum with shear. Scoliosis, tilting and rotation of the pelvis and contractures at the hips apply the load mainly on one ischial tuberosity or greater trochanter. Incontinence and sweating make the skin moist and prone to infection. Inability to speak and mental subnormality may diminish the frequency of attendance.

Uniform distribution of pressure, comfort and restful nights may be attained only by careful positioning in lying on a sheepskin on a pressure-relieving mattress with a pillow of polystyrene beads between the knees and a similar long cushion behind the trunk. Pain during the day from sitting askew and rotated, with almost all the weight borne on one buttock and thigh, with dislocated hip and separation of the legs for evacuation of the bladder and bowel, washing and drying demand one of two treatments. The first is conservative, employing seats which are individually made from sculptured polyurethane foam on plywood, a shapable matrix or a thermoplastic mould for sitting during the day and for defaecation, achieving the best position that is possible for comfort and function. The second involves surgical correction of the positions of the legs, pelvis and spine. Experience has grown in the last decade of pseudoarthroses at both hips and by resection of the proximal thirds of the femora (McCarthy *et al.*, 1988) and in the two-stage correction of spastic scoliosis by the implantation of Dwyer's wires by the anterior approach, followed by posterior instrumentation two weeks later. The results amply justify this major surgery and complications in lessening deformities, relieving pain, improving positioning and posture, and in gaining access to the perineum and facilitating transfers.

Stroke

This describes the sudden neurological defect caused either by haemorrhage into the brain or between the brain and skull or by ischaemia from occlusion of a cerebral artery by embolus or thrombosis. The incidence increases with age. The mental, motor and sensory disorders reflect the area of brain which is damaged and may conform to patterns of arterial supply. In the acute stage, unconsciousness, lying on a hard surface, immobility, anaesthesia and incontinence put at risk the skin over the sacrum, greater trochanters, heads of the fibulae, lateral malleoli and heels. A third of the patients die in three weeks and half are dead within a year. Damage within one cerebral hemisphere results in weakness or paralysis of the opposite side of the body, often accompanied by sensory deficiency or inattention. In the upper limb, spasticity affects principally the flexor muscles, and in the lower limb the extensor muscles, with the foot plantarflexed and inverted. This position of the foot, if uncorrected, causes the loads of the limb in sitting and of the body in standing to be borne on the lateral border of the forefoot. Through unrelieved pressure in lying or pressure of the boot or ill-fitting orthosis during the day the lateral malleolus too is prone to trophic ulceration.

Rheumatoid Arthritis

Causing chronic inflammation of the peripheral and central joints, the disease affects 1 per cent of the population and women twice more commonly then men and may begin at any age, but most often between 25 and 50 years. The cells lining the synovial membrane produce collagenases, interleukin 1 and prostaglandins, which may cause destruction of cartilage, subchondral bone, synovial capsule and ligaments. Deformities may develop rapidly, particularly flexion contractures. Instability of the cervical spine may cause myelopathy. The earlier that full treatment is instituted the better will be the prognosis. Despite adequate rest, exercise, analgesic anti-inflammatory drugs, protection of damaged joints, gold, penicillamine, suphasalazine, corticosteroids, immunosuppressant drugs and surgery, 5 to 10 per cent of patients become severely disabled. Through changes in dermal collagen, splitting of elastic fibres, thinning of subcutaneous tissues and vasculitis skin is friable and heals slowly, all aggravated by corticosteroid treatment. Moreover chronic anaemia, reduced mobility and diminished nutrition may come later and pressure sores may accelerate death.

Diabetes Mellitus

This features abnormal insulin secretion, fasting hyperglycaemia, decreased glucose tolerance, large-vessel disease, microvascular disease and neuropathy. The elevation of blood glucose and alteration of lipid metabolism are caused by relative or absolute lack of insulin secretion with excess of circulating stress hormones. Large-vessel disease is common: atherosclerosis in the intima and calcification in the media of arterial walls coming more frequently, at an earlier age and more severely in diabetics. About 30 per cent of all diabetics eventually develop peripheral vascular disease and lower-limb amputations are 5 times more frequent in those who have diabetes. In microvascular disease the basement membrane in the capillaries of skin, skeletal muscle, kidneys, pancreas, heart and nervous system is thickened. The longer diabetes mellitus is present the more likely is serious vascular disease. In sensory and motor peripheral nerves, nerve roots, autonomic nerves and the spinal cord there is focal degeneration of myelin and Schwann cells. Sensori-motor polyneuropathy is the most frequent form of diabetic neuropathy, often presenting as painless penetrating ulcers on the sole of the foot.

PROPHYLAXIS

In all these diseases tissues may break down unless preventive measures are taken: prevention demands priority; there is no better treatment. The prevalence of grade 2, 3 and 4 sores, i.e. all but the most superficial abrasions, in hospital patients ranges in different surveys from 3 per cent (Petersen and Bittman, 1971) to 8.8 per cent (Barbenel *et al.*, 1977). A prevalence of 5 per cent would mean that at any one time 30 000 patients in British hospitals have at least one definite pressure sore, indicating the level of breakdown in patient care.

There are six precepts for the prevention of pressure sores.

1. Recognise those who are at risk. Most pressure sores develop within 2 weeks of the admission of patients to hospital and preventive action begins at the moment of admission if not before. The risk factors and the rating scales have been discussed in Chapters 3 and 5. The completion of the rating takes less than a minute, yet, most regrettably, such a simple and rapid assessment on admission and thereafter weekly is not practised routinely in every hospital and nursing home. If it were, and if appropriate action followed, the majority of pressure sores would be prevented (Amies *et al.*, 1980).
2. Distribute weight evenly and over the widest surface area of the body that is practicable. Different materials exist for supporting patients in bed. The merits of the materials and the various support systems are discussed in Chapters 7 and 18. The choice can be the patient's after trial, judged by comfort, ability to relax, quality and duration of sleep,

fewer calls for attention during the night, reduced sedation and analgesia and expressed satisfaction.

3. Change the patient's position at 2-hourly intervals. The exact time that pressure can be tolerated before injury begins is uncertain because the intrinsic determinants are crucial, inter-related and variable. The practice of 2-hourly turning has proved to be effective in reducing the incidence of sores and this period is hallowed by tradition. Kosiak (1961) showed with an animal model that a pressure of only 70 mmHg (9.3 kPa) applied constantly for 2 hours produced irreversible tissue damage but not if pressure were intermittently relieved. In hospital and in the community, equipment for the prevention of pressure sores must play an increasing role with nursing skills deployed in recognising the patients at high risks and in delivering specialised care. When wards are staffed at night by a maximum of two nurses 2-hourly turning of a patient is only occasionally possible. Manual turning may be replaced by turning and lateral tilting beds such as the LIC Turnover Bed (Power-Tech Ltd, West Sussex), although its mattress is relatively hard. Net suspension beds, such as the one manufactured by Egerton (Egerton Hospital Equipment Ltd, Horsham) have not found universal favour and do not give good support for the spine.

   A person sitting for long in a wheelchair, even sitting on a pressure-relieving cushion, should if possible lift the buttocks clear from the seat every 10 to 15 minutes by pushing down on the propelling wheels or armrests. Paraplegic patients learn to perform push-ups and tetraplegics relieve pressure by leaning to one side or the other. An alternating pressure seat cushion (BASE, Talley Equipment Ltd, Borehamwood) was designed with the same objective. There are many different wheelchair cushions available and the choice is made by trial and individual preference guided by measurements of interface pressures, aiming at pressures under 40 mmHg (5.3 kPa). Slashing polyurethane foam into cubes for most of the depth of the cushion allows compression of the cubes separately without surface limitation.

4. All skin surfaces which bear load should be thoroughly inspected in a good light at least once every day for redness or induration. Whether people can look after themselves or must rely upon others, the routine of daily visual inspection and palpation for the earliest signs of tissue damage must never be broken. Fastidious skin care is especially necessary when there is neurological defect.

5. Skin should be kept clean and dry to prevent maceration, especially in the perineum, groins and natal cleft, and over the buttocks and thighs. Damp skin breaks down more easily under axial pressure and shear forces. Contiguous skin surfaces under large folds should be kept separated by fluffed cotton wool or sausage-shaped polystyrene bead cushions. Resilient natural sheepskin is pre-eminent in the absorption

of water vapour and this quality above others accounts for its major contribution in preventing pressure sores. Water vapour can be removed from the interface by ventilation and by absorption. Vapour absorption is the dominant mechanism and much more effective than ventilation in maintaining a low-humidity interface (Denne, 1979). In a saturated atmosphere at 30 °C, natural sheepskin was shown to absorb 15 times more water vapour than a polyester simulation. Soiled or wet clothes and incontinence pads should be changed without delay. Bedclothes should be changed frequently, using sheets which are soft, clean and free from wrinkles. Draw sheets should not be used because they can increase both shear forces and interface pressures. In fever and hot weather the skin should be sponged and washed often and dried gently and thoroughly. Talcum powder should be applied only sparingly and not at all in skin folds.

6. Activity should be encouraged and passive, assisted and resisted exercises performed. Over-sedation should be avoided because immobility surpasses all other causes of pressure sores. Movements change the pressure, ventilation, humidity and temperature at the interface. Paraplegics learn the importance of the discipline of push-ups and for those who need insistent reminders, alarms based on time and change in pressure have been developed, with automatic reset when the seat pressure is relieved (Chawla *et al.*, 1978). The majority retain the habit of lifting effectively but lapse in frequency, continuing to need 10-minute reminders.

Technical Aids to Prevention

With the singular exception of shear, all extrinsic factors in the genesis of trophic ulcers can be measured. A package of sensors is required to judge who is at risk. The thresholds for pressure, temperature, humidity, pH and time will be determined individually and pre-set. When any threshold is reached an audible or visual warning will indicate when the position must be changed. The foundation will be a pressure-monitoring system, such as the Oxford Pressure Monitor, described in Chapter 17, to which other sensors will be added. This pressure monitor has become a standard tool for orthotists, engineers, therapists and plaster technicians. It is in daily use in the technical and functional evaluations of supporting surfaces, and measuring interface pressures in the conservative management of paralytic, idiopathic and spastic scoliosis by spinal braces (Chase *et al.*, 1989). It has also been used in the manufacture of individual seating for severely disabled people for whom no standard seat and accessories have sufficed. For them a thermoplastic moulded seat (Figure 8.1), shapable matrix body

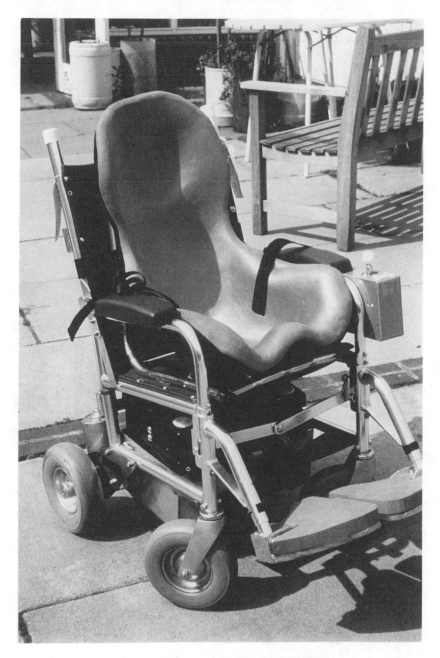

Figure 8.1 Thermoplastic moulded seat

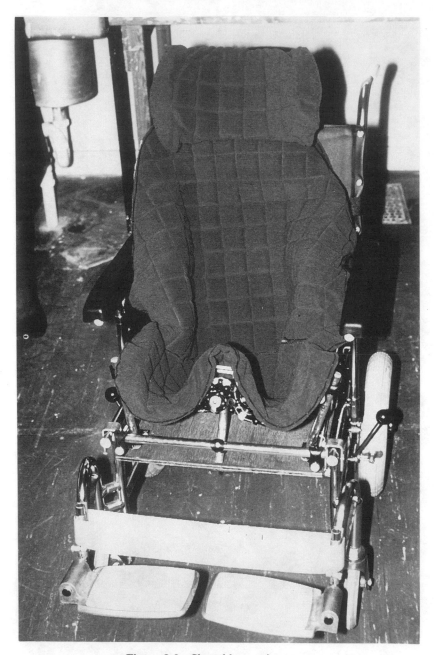

Figure 8.2   Shapable matrix seat

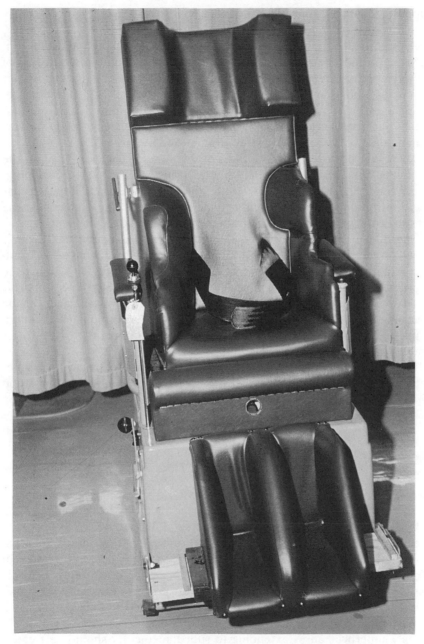

Figure 8.3 Seat constructed of sculptured foam on a plywood base, covered in polyvinylchloride with cotton backing

support (Figure 8.2) or sculptured foam on plywood base (Figure 8.3) may be necessary.

A thermoplastic mould is made in four stages (McQuilton and Johnson, 1981). The most favourable sitting position is obtained on a soft bag of polystyrene beads which is then consolidated by vacuum; a positive plaster cast is made and on the refined cast heated plastazote (BXL Plastics Ltd, Manningtree) is drape-formed, and then supporting that a rigid thermoplastic outer shell is formed in the same way; the finished moulded support is mounted on a tubular aluminium frame to fit in a wheelchair.

There are, however, disadvantages of this system. The close fit limits the person to one position and may hinder transfer. The plastazote lining, which retains heat and impedes ventilation, can wear out and if the cast has not been retained the entire seat may need renewal. Any change in shape or size of the person may necessitate the production of a new seat.

The matrix body support (Cousins *et al.*, 1982) is constructed from a sheet of interlinked plastic and metal parts held together by ball-and-socket joints, which allow movement of the components for shaping the support. The shape is then retained by tightening the joints. The support is lined by quilted foam upholstery, which is easily removed and can be machine-washed, and the finished seat is mounted on a tubular aluminium frame to fit in a wheelchair. Headrest, armrests, footrests, tray, harness and lap straps are added as required.

Individually sculptured foam seats are made of approved flame-retardant foam cut and assembled piecemeal to achieve optimal position and glued together onto a plywood frame and covered overall by a cotton or woollen fabric.

TREATMENT OF AN ESTABLISHED PRESSURE SORE

Like an iceberg, the ulcer has a small visible surface and an extensive unknown base. There are few non-invasive methods of determining the extent, such as the one described in Chapter 13, but the size of the diseased area can be shown by X-rays (Figure 8.4), ultrasound scanning, sinogram or magnetic resonance imaging. Pressure obliterates blood vessels in muscle more readily than in dermis and subcutaneous fat, and when soft tissue is compressed against bone the highest pressure is close to the bone. Necrotic muscle liquefies and if it becomes infected the abscess must be drained.

Only superficial sores extending to subcutaneous fat should be treated conservatively, keeping the area exposed, free from pressure, clean and moist. The responsibility for nursing care, it is generally accepted, rests with the sister in charge of the ward, and commonly this extends to the choice of the bed or mattress and prescription for the sore. Attention

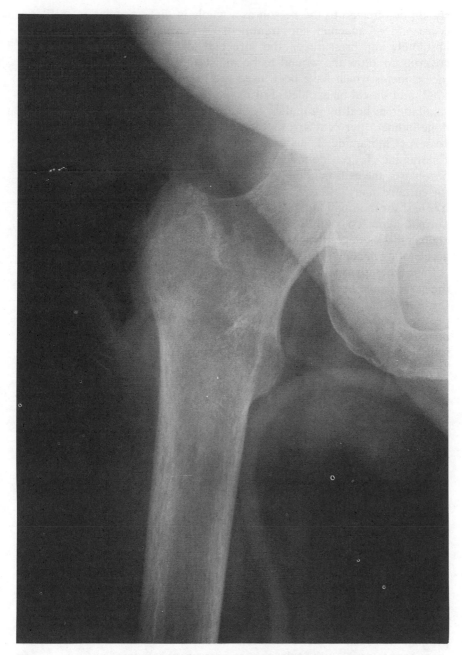

Figure 8.4 Radiograph showing a large flask-shaped cavity and osteomyelitis of the greater trochanter in a woman suffering from multiple sclerosis, with urinary incontinence managed by an indwelling catheter

should be directed to the person as a whole in diet, stimulation, activity, correction of anaemia and treatment of concurrent illnesses, refusing absolutely any pressure on the sore and ideally providing a protective covering to allow the wound to be moist and undisturbed. Many of the medicaments which have been used are harmful (Cameron and Leaper, 1987) and should be avoided. For example, Eusol and chloramine T close capillaries in healthy granulation tissue never to be reopened and povi-done-iodine 5 per cent arrests blood flow in all but the largest capillary vessels. Chloramine T disrupts collagen synthesis and delays healing. Chloramine T, povidone-iodine and hydrogen peroxide are toxic to fibroblasts, the cells in granulation tissue which lay down collagen. Behind the curtains many different lotions are applied and it should be known that it is best for the small ulcer to be left undisturbed, except for cleaning with normal saline. To combine absorbancy with moist wound healing, calcium alginate is biodegradable and provides absorption without adherence, accelerating healing (Thomas, 1985).

Physiotherapy is vital to the treatment of the whole person in encouraging movements. In particular it can increase the power in use of the parts of the body that are under voluntary control, in passive movements to prevent contractures, in functional activities, ventilation of the lungs and effective coughing but no longer in treating the ulcer. Ice, ultraviolet rays, ionised steam, ultrasound, pulsed high-frequency energy, laser therapy and massage have been advocated and practised (Fernandez, 1988; Dyson and Suckling, 1978). However, superficial wounds heal better undisturbed under absorbent protective dressings. There is a need to compare the efficacy of these physical treatment modalities using controlled clinical trials.

More extensive wounds need surgical treatment. When the defect is small and the surrounding tissues can be mobilized, direct closure may be possible. If there is necrosis extending to muscle a surgeon's advice should be sought early about debridement and reconstruction. Necrotic tissue should be removed by forceps and scissors. The fibrous capsule of an established diseased area may be completely excised. If there is bone in the base of the ulcer, diseased bone should be removed in entirety and any bone in the base of the ulcer which by prominence may predispose to further tissue necrosis by pressure should be reduced by the removal of a 15 mm sliver. Closure of extensive wounds may be delayed for the formation of healthy granulation tissue. Reconstruction may be achieved later by a sliding full-thickness skin flap graft, especially over large bony prominences such as the trochanters, ischia and sacrum, since scar tissue there cannot develop the tolerance to pressure that is needed.

Wet dressings of normal saline should be used. In a moist, uninfected environment within 3 days a layer of granulation tissue forms over newly exposed viable tissue, but if the exposed surface dries secondary desiccation necrosis occurs under a coagulum. Concentrated antiseptics carry double risks of inducing additional necrosis and retarding granulation tissue. Dressings should keep the wound moist, avoid pooling of pus, and contour to the wound surface without preventing contraction. Tight packing must be avoided, oxygen diffusion must be allowed and non-absorbable particles must not be shed. The dry beads of Debrisan (trademark of a dextran polymer glucose, Pharmacia Ltd, Milton Keynes) may be used for indolent ulcers and in taking up exudate to four times the initial weight the polymer slowly hydrates to form a gel and expands. There are new hydrophilic polymers and calcium alginate gel, Sorbsan (NI Medical Ltd, Redditch), is preferred. Silicone rubber foam, which is cast by pouring into a diseased area, can be removed, washed and replaced when the wound is cleaned with normal saline once or twice daily and is renewed as the wound contracts.

Currently, pressure sores are costing the National Health Service at least £250 million annually, yet this immense medical, social and economic millstone is not inescapable. This figure can be drastically reduced if three conditions are met: first, if infirm and disabled people and those who look after them at home, in nursing homes and in hospitals are unceasingly alert and ever mindful of the dangers; second, if they are determined on prevention by seeking out those at risk and ensuring that they receive care in their general health and move, or are moved as much as possible – 'where there is no pressure, there is no sore'; and third, if in hospital and in the community emphasis and money switches from treatment to prevention, ensuring alertness and that the right equipment is at hand.

REFERENCES

Amies, A., Chiarcossi, A. and Jiminez, J. (1980). Management of pressure sores. Comparative study in medical and surgical patients. *Postgrad. Med.*, **67**, 177–182

Barbenel, J. C., Jordan, M. M., Nichol, S. M. and Clark, M. (1977). The incidence of pressure sores in the Greater Glasgow Health Board. *Lancet*, **ii**, 548–550

Cameron, S. and Leaper, D. (1987). Antiseptic toxicity in open wounds. *Care, Science and Practice*, **5** (2), 19–20

Chase, A. P., Bader, D. L. and Houghton, G. (1989). The biomechanical effectiveness of the Boston Brace in the management of adolescent idiopathic scoliosis. *Spine*, **14**(6), 636–642.

Chawla, J. C., Andrews, B. and Bar, C. (1978). Using warning devices to improve pressure-relief training. *Paraplegia*, **16**, 413–419

Cousins, S. J., Jones, K. N. and Ackerley, K. E. (1982). Contoured cushion fabrication. *Care, Science and Practice*, **1** (3), 15–18

Denne, W. A. (1979). An objective assessment of the sheepskins used for decubitus sore prevention. *Rheum. and Rehabil.*, **18**, 23–29

Dyson, M. and Suckling, J. (1978). Stimulation of tissue repair by ultrasound. A survey of the mechanics involved. *Physiotherapy*, **64** (4), 105–108

Fernandez, S. (1988). Prevention and treatment of pressure sores. *Care, Science and Practice*, **6** (1), 17–21

Kosiak, M. (1961). Etiology of decubitus ulcers. *Arch. Phys. Med. Rehabil.*, **42**, 83–89

McCarthy, R. E., Simon, S., Douglas, B., Zawacki, R. and Reese, N. (1988). Proximal femoral resection to allow adults who have severe cerebral palsy to sit. *J. Bone Joint Surg.*, **70A**, 1011–1016

McQuilton, G. and Johnson, G. R. (1981). Cost effective moulded seating for the handicapped child. *Pros. Orthop. Int.*, **5**, 37–41

Petersen, N. C. and Bittman, S. (1971). The epidemiology of pressure sores. *Scand. J. Plast. Reconstr. Surg.*, **5**, 62–66

Thomas, S. (1985). Use of a calcium alginate dressing. *Pharmaceutical J.*, **235**, 188–190

9

Spinal Injury

J. R. Silver

HISTORICAL BACKGROUND

Pressure sores have been known since antiquity; their association with the disease of nervous system was first suggested in 1593 by Fabricius, who implicated severance of peripheral nerves. There were a series of accounts by Bright (1821) and Brodie (1836) who described their evolution in patients with traumatic injuries of the spinal cord. However it is to Charcot (1877) that we owe the first scientific analysis of the causation of pressure sores, in a very full description of the pathogenesis of sores in diseases of the spinal cord and of the nervous system. His work was seminal, and as it has either been ignored or misquoted it is worthwhile studying his concepts in detail. He stressed that the causation of the sore in cerebral and spinal cases was the same, that anaesthesia of the paralysed part was not the sole cause, and that the patient with incomplete lesions also got sores. He recognised that rapid atrophy of the tissues contributed, as did immobility. He also recognised the role of pressure but considered it secondary. He tried to alleviate this by turning the patient regularly. He stressed that sores could appear in two days and carried an ominous prognosis, and indeed called them 'ominous' sores.

When an acute bed-sore appears under the influence of a lesion of the spinal cord, it shows itself in the very great majority of cases in the sacral region and consequently above and internal to the chosen seat of eschars of cerebral origin. Here it occupies the median line and extends symmetrically, on either side, towards the adjacent parts. It may, indeed, happen that only one side will be affected. In the case, for instance, where a lateral half of the cord is alone engaged then the cutaneous lesion frequently shows itself on the opposite side of the body from the spinal lesion.

The influence of attitudes here plays an important part. Thus it is customary when the patients are so placed as to repose on the side, during part of the day, to find, besides the sacral eschar, vast necrosive ulcerations developing on the trochanteric regions. It is also common enough to see, contrary to what happens in cerebral cases, that the different parts of the paralysed limbs which are exposed to even slight and brief pressure, as the ankles, heels and inner surface of the knees, present lesions characteristic of an acute bed-sore. Eschars may also show themselves, but indeed very rarely, on a level with the apex of the scapula, or over the olecranon process.

Speaking generally, we may say that the spinal lesions which produce acute bed-sores are also those which give rise to rapid muscular atrophy and to other disorders of the same class. The almost simultaneous development of these different consecutive affections makes it seem probable, already, that they have a common origin. (Charcot, 1877.)

He stressed that they were infected and dangerous and they commonly gave rise to fever in the acute stage, relapsing fever in the chronic stage. They gave rise to a spread of infection and dissemination of septic emboli. He made minute descriptions of the superficial vesicular eruption and of the underlying tumorification and cellulitis of the tissue. He was aware of the dangers of maceration of the skin caused by continuous seepage of urine, which he tried to avoid by means of intermittent catheterisation.

He noted that paralysis of the sympathetic nervous system could give rise to hyperaemia and a raised peripheral temperature of the tissues, but he did not believe that this retarded healing, quite the contrary.

It is the role of trophic nerves that is most widely misquoted and misunderstood, and Charcot (1877) interpreted them in the following words:

... before adopting a theory which cannot subsist without calling out a whole system of nerves whose existence is as yet problematical, it is necessary to make sure, by every means, that it is really impossible to explain the phenomena, the interpretation of which is required, by appealing to the properties of the different nerves already known. We must take care not to infringe the axiom of Logic, '*Haud multiplicanda entia absque necessitate.*' ['One must take care not to multiply more entities than necessity dictates.'] Now, the vasomotor theory being eliminated, there yet undoubtedly remains much to be done from this point of view [Figure 9.1].

Subsequent to the work of Charcot there was little written about pressure sores in paraplegic patients. Patients died rapidly from the complications of sores or from urinary infections and the subsequent descriptions were mainly devoted to the pathological consequences. Thompson Walker (1917, 1937) found that of 397 patients with spinal injuries admitted to the King George V Military Hospital, 47 per cent died from urinary tract complications within 8 to 10 weeks of injury. Later, both in the United States and in the United Kingdom (Munro, 1945, 1947; Holdsworth, 1963; Guttmann, 1976) it was shown that by admitting patients rapidly to specialised centres and with regular turning and the correct treatment of the bladder, pressure sores could be prevented and established pressure sores healed up.

Sir Ludwig Guttman's pioneering work heralded the modern era of pressure sore management. It is reviewed by Guttmann (1953 and 1976), and there is now established literature, of which this book is an example, on all aspects of pressure sores, although this chapter will deal with those specific aspects that are different in paraplegic patients.

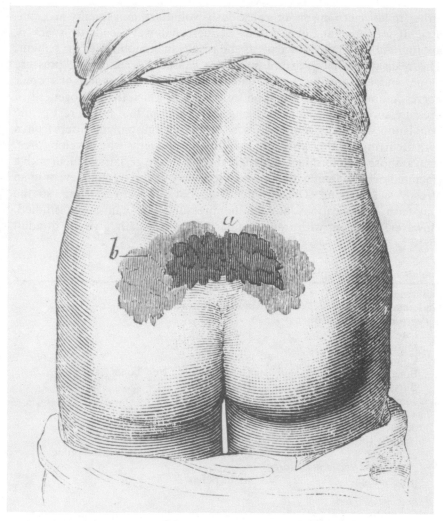

Figure 9.1   Pressure sore from Charcot's textbook

PATHOGENESIS

It is accepted that the basis of a pressure sore is continuous, unrelieved pressure. When pressure is exerted upon normally innervated tissue, painful stimuli arise that are transmitted centrally. These sensations are received by the peripheral receptors and are transmitted via the sensory nerves to the spinal cord. Spinal reflex movement is elicited. Alternatively, the sensations may be transmitted through to the higher centres where either reflex mechanisms or consciously voluntary movements are initiated. It follows that injury to any of these pathways leads to a lack of appropriate protecting movements and results in immobility of the patient. The realisation that pressure sores are caused by continuing pressure alone, and are not due to the damage of specific vasomotor or trophic nerves, tended to divert attention from ways in which the pathogenesis of pressure sores in paraplegic patients differed from that in the rest of the population. However, a pressure sore in a paraplegic patient differs from a sore occurring in other groups at risk. In other patients who develop sores, such as those with terminal malignant disease or the geriatric patient with a fractured neck of femur, the pressure sore may be the terminal event in an already sick patient. These patients do not survive very long, so the long-term complications due to the pressure sore cannot be studied. However, a patient with traumatic paraplegia is usually a young fit adult

Table 9.1   Acute complications of pressure sores

Failure to heal	
Undermining tissues *locally* and at a *distance* through tissue planes	
Penetration of deep tissues	
Fat	Fat necrosis
Muscle	Muscle necrosis
Connective tissue	Fourniers gangerene
Bone	Osteomyelitis New bone
Bursa	Bursitis
Joints	Septic arthritis
For example: *ischial sore*	
penetrates	to the pelvis and ischial ramus sinuses
laterally (posteriorly)	to the hip (knee) joint
anteriorly	to the groin when patient nursed prone
trochanteric sore	
penetrates	to the pelvis
All sores are infected	
Celllullitis	
Gangerene	
Systemic effects	
Septicaemia	
Acute ulcerative	
endocarditis	
Nutritional	Loss of appetite
	Emaciation
	Acute and low grade flare-ups with temperature
	Malaise
Psychological	Acute febrile confusional state leading to possible depression and/or aggression
Smell	Effect upon relatives and patient

who, once the initial injury has been treated, can return home to an active life. However, continued anaesthesia puts the skin at risk of developing pressure sores throughout life and any sores developed can give rise to long-term complications. The immediate consequences of pressure sores, their complications and long-term effects cannot be adequately dealt with in one chapter. For reference purposes, they are summarised in Tables 9.1 to 9.4.

There has been a dearth of information on the long-term consequences of sores. Little research has been carried out on such simple matters as the incidence, the size and the depth of the sore. Attention in the past has been directed at the sore and the idea that this was a breakdown of tissue rather than at the concept that it was a breakdown of the caring system. Thus we

Table 9.2 Complications of chronic pressure sores

Chronic discharging sinus
Sequestra formation
Amyloid disease
Any of the acute complications

Table 9.3 Complications of healed sores

Scar tissue	Inelastic
	Damage
Adherence to bone	Does not move
	Shear
Atrophy of subcutaneous tissue	
Cosmetic	
Ectopic bone	Contracture – loss of mobility

Table 9.4 Distant effects of pressure sores

Effects of immobilisation in bed	
Psychological	Depression at stoppage of treatment
	Realisation of significance of body – that it is not your servant but your master
Retention of urine	
Constipation	
Increase of spasticity	
Pneumonia	In dependent side – due to immobilisation in bed
Contractures	In parts of body away from the sore – hips, knees, feet
Shoulder–hand syndrome	
Amyloid disease	

must look at why, where and how a patient gets sores, what are the economic and sociological consequences of sores, and what are the long-term effects.

Why Do Patients Develop Pressure Sores Immediately after Sustaining Spinal Injury?

The majority of traumatic spinal injuries are caused by road traffic accidents, falls or industrial accidents, and 75 per cent of them are accompanied by multiple trauma. Silver *et al.* (1980) looked at a consecutive series of 100 patients with acute traumatic spinal injuries. Fifty had severe head injuries and so were unable to co-operate, 27 had fractured extremities and 32 had fractured ribs with chest injuries. The patient was generally in a shocked state from blood loss, so lowering of the blood pressure and tissue oxygen with reduction in the perfusion pressure was apparent. They were admitted to the local receiving hospital and only transferred to a spinal centre after a period, usually when their life-threatening complications had been treated. Unfortunately, by this time they may have acquired severe pressure sores that delayed the rehabilita-

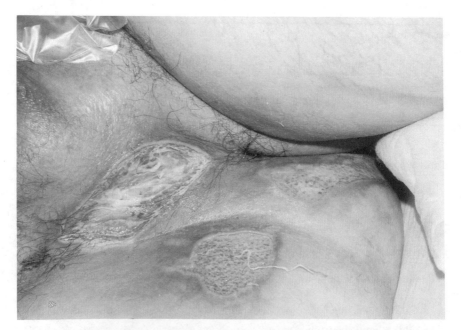

Figure 9.2 Pressure sore caused by Thomas splint in paraplegic patient with a fractured lower limb

tion by many months. Silver (1975) found in one series of 57 acute spinal injuries admitted to a spinal centre that 20 had pressure sores, an incidence of 35 per cent. In 1981 Richardson and Meyer found that 134 out of 180 patients admitted to a spinal centre 72 hours after injury had sores, in contrast to no observed sores in the 122 patients admitted within 72 hours.

The various causes of pressure sore development are most conveniently listed as follows:

1. The management of the associated injuries, such as fracture of the extremity, may well cause pressure sores; misuse of the equipment, e.g. Thomas splints (Figure 9.2) and unpadded plaster-of-Paris casts, also gives rise to sores, as they are unsuitable for use with an anaesthetic leg. There may be priority given to the management of the chest via drains and the patient is not turned in consequence (Figure 9.3).
2. There will be a lowering of the blood pressure by sympathetic paralysis, with a loss of vasomotor reflexes even in the absence of surgical shock.
3. Prolonged lying on an operating or X-ray table or in a casualty department can cause pressure sores.
4. There may be a lack of understanding of the management of spinal fractures. There is a correct fear that injudicious movement of the fractured spine can increase neurological deficit so the patients are not moved at all, and unfortunately the normal regime of nursing patients in a general hospital is to let the patient lie flat on his or her back without being turned. There is a misguided view that the patient has to be transported as quickly as possible to the spinal unit, so that no special measures are required to treat the patient. There are also misguided ideas about the management of spinal fractures, so the patient may well be immobilised by rods or corseted and sat up immediately while still in the shocked state or in pain, with the result that they sit slumped in pain in the chair or in a plaster-of-Paris jacket (Figure 9.4). The dangers in normal people of prolonged recumbancy have been long recognised and they are greater in a paralysed patient.
5. Spinal fractures may not be diagnosed at all. Regrettably, spinal injuries not accompanied by total paralysis are frequently missed, owing to an associated head injury. Alternatively, the diagnosis is made only when the patient is retained of urine and has developed deep pressure sores.

In one British regional spinal injuries centre it was found (Cook, 1961) that of 70 tetraplegic patients half were referred without the lesion being identified. A systematic study of a consecutive series of 353 traumatic spinal injury patients, admitted under the care of one consultant, showed that the injury of the spinal cord had not been recognised at the receiving hospital in 15 cases, and that in at least 10 cases mis-diagnosis of the cord injury resulted in significant neurological deterioration (Ravichandran and Silver, 1982). The contributory factors

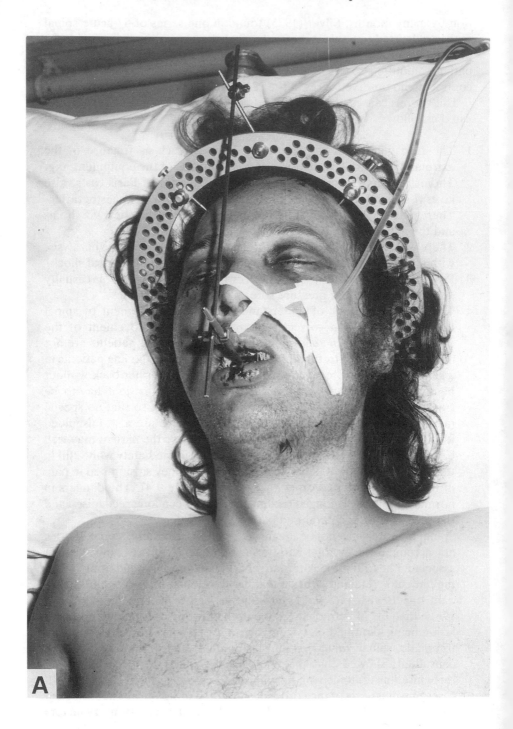

A

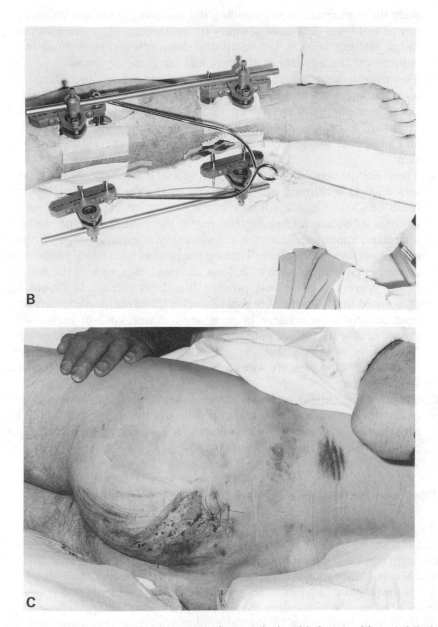

Figure 9.3 Patient sustained a traumatic paraplegia with fractured jaw and limb and laceration of his buttocks in a road accident. Treatment of the fractures was totally unsuited to a paraplegic patient because regular turning was unsuitable, with disastrous consequences upon the skin

were the circumstances surrounding the accident, the initial absence of
any neurological deficit, head injury or suppression of consciousness by
drugs, multiple injuries, radiographical diagnostic errors, and failure to
apppreciate the mechanism of injury and the causes involved.

6. The overall situation may well be compounded by the effects of
malnutrition. Since in the first few days following a spinal injury patients
suffer from paralytic ileus and are unable to tolerate food by mouth and
are likely to be nourished on intravenous saline, antibiotics, steroids
and analgesics. None of these drugs can improve the nutrition of the
skin.

7. There is also a misplaced confidence in special equipment. Although the
introduction of turning beds, large-cell mattresses and striker frames
has been a considerable advance in the prevention of pressure sores, it
is not a substitute for regular turning of the patient and the medical
attendants cannot abdicate the responsibility of ensuring regular turns
carried out around the clock. Turning the patient must be supplemented
by proper equipment, such as pillows and sand bags, to hold the patient
in the correct position and prevent him from rolling. It should be
recognised that with the shortage of nurses there may well be only one
inadequately trained nurse on a general duties ward at night, who
cannot ensure that all the patients are attended to and turned regularly.
It is hardly surprising that the patients who are admitted to general
hospitals develop pressure sores unless they are rapidly transferred to a
spinal centre.

8. The standard nursing regime is often inadequate. The hammock effect
of the draw sheet, caustic washing powder on the sheets and failure to
turn the patient regularly are all causes of sores on any patients at risk in
a hospital, in particular the spinal patient.

The Reason for Developing Pressure Sores at a Spinal Centre

It is easy to be critical of general hospitals that do not have proper facilities
and the knowledge of how to treat spinal injury patients, but regrettably
pressure sores do occur in spinal centres. In the United States, Richardson
and Meyer (1981) analysed a group of 122 patients who were admitted to a
spinal unit within 72 hours of injury. None of these patients had pressure
sores on admission to hospital. However, 81 patients developed sores while
under treatment because of the misguided view that the skin could be
neglected while the spinal cord was looked after. In other words, the
cutaneous system was always superseded by the central nervous (brain),
cardiorespiratory, gastrointestinal, genitourinary and the musculoskeletal
systems in these multiple, systemic trauma patients. With appropriate
surgical and medical treatments and stabilisation of these other systems,

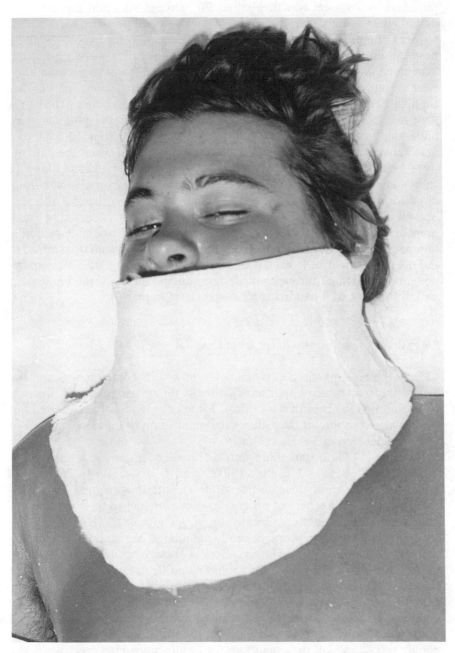

Figure 9.4 Patient with acute injury of the cervical spine from diving in the Mediterranean area. He was flown back to the UK in this state. The plaster of Paris did not immobilise the spine and certainly did not help the skin

the cutaneous system was then cared for. Thyagarajan and Silver (1984) described 25 acutely injured patients who developed pressure sores within 5 weeks of injury. Twenty-three of these patients developed sores while in hospital and 2 while on weekend leave. All the sores were superficial. Seventeen of these were in women who developed sacral sores when they were being mobilized and were undergoing a programme of bladder training. This type of sore did not occur in male patients. The sores developed in the early stages of rehabilitation when the patients were undergoing bladder training. Quite specifically, urine trickled back and macerated the skin. The remaining sores also occurred when the patients were being mobilized and were due to unsuitable or tight clothing (2 cases), improperly fitting calipers (2), burns (1) and the excessive abnormal bone formation around the joints (3). This was due to the fact the skin became adherent to the bone. The author has also observed a small number of deeper sores. These have occurred when there has been a failure of specific equipment, or when the patients have been transferred to the operating theatre. It is vital that trained members of staff accompany patients at all stages throughout the hospital and also that the equipment and trolleys are well padded at all stages (see Chapter 6).

Sores that Develop on Discharge from Hospital

Clearly the level of the neurological lesion and its completeness and the age of the patient are important factors in the development of pressure sores, but it is the care that is critical. Little research has been carried out on this aspect. Some of the failures that contribute to the development of sores are detailed in Tables 9.3 and 9.4.

Between 1947 and 1967 there were 141 cases of traumatic tetraplegia at the Liverpool Regional Centre (Silver and Gibbon, 1968). When the patients had finished their course of treatment the majority were discharged home, but others of no greater disability had to be discharged to long-term accommodation, usually on social grounds. The fate of the severely paralysed tetraplegic depended to a large degree on social factors and only to a limited degree on the physical extent of their paralysis. When there was a devoted relative the patient could be discharged home, while those not in this fortunate position were discharged to a long-term hostel or hospital. Of the 29 patients discharged to hospital or hostel, 13 died; by comparison, of the 79 discharged home only 10 died. Patients discharged home were looked after by at least one full-time person and what these people lacked in skill they made up for in affection. However, when the patient was admitted to long-term accommodation, the long-term nursing care that was available was equivalent to about 1 hour a day and this was not sufficient to keep a tetraplegic in good health.

A further analysis was made of patients readmitted with sores to the National Spinal Injuries Centre who had been initially discharged home fit and free of sores (Thyagarajan and Silver, 1984). In these 75 patients there were two peaks; one of these occurred within 1 year of discharge (19 sores), followed by a scattering of sores until a further peak occurred at 10 to 15 years. Sores that occurred within the first year of discharge were due to many factors. For example, the patients had not been adequately taught how to look after themselves at the hospital. Other patients rejected their injury on psychological grounds or were not prepared to make any compromise to looking after their body, or were unable to owing to brain injuries. Once patients had passed through this difficult time and either succumbed to their sores or learned to look after themselves, the number of sores decreased and the patients remained relatively well until a second peak when the sores occurred at 10–15 years. This phase may have occurred as attendant care broke down and the patients themselves were ageing. It may also have been associated with the patients developing problems of arthritis of their shoulders, ascending syringomyelocele, urinary tract infection and obesity, so that self-care became impossible.

The risk of pressure sores occurring was the commonest cause through-out life of the patient being readmitted to hospital. In a study of 100 spinal patients, sores constituted 15 per cent of readmissions (Creek *et al.*, 1987). The occurrence of these sores can be reduced by a peripatetic nursing service, regular check-ups, chair and cushion clinics at the parent spinal unit and by admitting these patients to appropriate local facilities for short-term relief for the families. This clearly requires specialized relief services at the local disability unit. It is less than helpful to admit these spinal patients to the local orthopaedic or geriatric wards, since they do not possess adequate trained staff to look after the patients and need the facilities for their own acute admissions. Eight patients developed sores who had been free of them when admitted to the local hospital for social leave when relatives became ill.

THE LONG-TERM EFFECTS OF PRESSURE SORES

Virtually all the information about pressure sores in paraplegic patients is hospital based, relating to severe sores that have required hospital admission. Little information is known about the epidemiology of pressure sores in the community. Even such a dramatic event as death and its relationship to pressure sores is not known outside the hospital population, owing to the inadequate information on the death certificate and the difficulty in patient follow-up. The most comprehensive work in this field has been performed in Canada by Breithaupt, Jousse and Geisler in a series of papers between 1961 and 1983. They followed up all the patients at their centre. They found that of 1909 identified patients, 428 were known to be dead and of these 19, that is 4.4 per cent, died of pressure sores. There is, in contrast, very full information about the patients who died in hospital, and while the septic effects of pressure sores are quite apparent in the acute stage, the long-term effects are little appreciated, possibly because the patient died from overwhelming sepsis and did not survive.

However, in the paraplegic population there is a unique opportunity to study the long-term effects of pressure sores. However, it must be appreciated that the hospital population is a selected population and only certain paraplegic patients are admitted to hospital and have died there and have had post-mortems carried out. The largest series is that of Tribe and Silver (1969) who carried out a study of the post-mortems at the National Spinal Injuries Centre between 1944 and 1965. There were 220 post-mortems, of whom 174 died more than three months after injury. This work was continued to include a further 214 post-mortems carried out up to 1980 of whom 155 died more than three months after injury (Baker *et al.*, 1984). The incidence of amyloidosis was extraordinarily similar in the two groups; 65 patients in the former series and 61 cases in the latter. These patients died predominantly from renal failure. The organs chiefly involved were kidneys, liver and spleen. No cases were found among the acute paraplegic patients and all the cases included histological confirmation. The two most important aetiological factors causing amyloid disease were pressure sores and urinary tract infections. Previous literature suggested that pressure sores with underlying osteomyelitis were the chief factors in producing amyloidosis in paraplegia. For this reason, the incidence of pressure sores and osteomyelitis was studied in these patients. The sites and severity of the pressure sores were reported in the clinical notes, but the true incidence of underlying osteomyelitis could be assessed only by studying the X-rays. Of the patients in the Tribe series with amyloidosis, 60 had severe pressure sores and in 47 of these there was radiological or operative evidence of underlying osteomyelitis (Figure 9.5). The findings in the Baker series were almost identical. Renal sepsis alone could not cause amyloid.

Clinical Manifestations of Amyloidosis

The chief effects are the result of kidney involvement, with the patients presenting with a nephrotic syndrome.

Oedema

This is the most striking clinical manifestation of amyloidosis in paraplegic

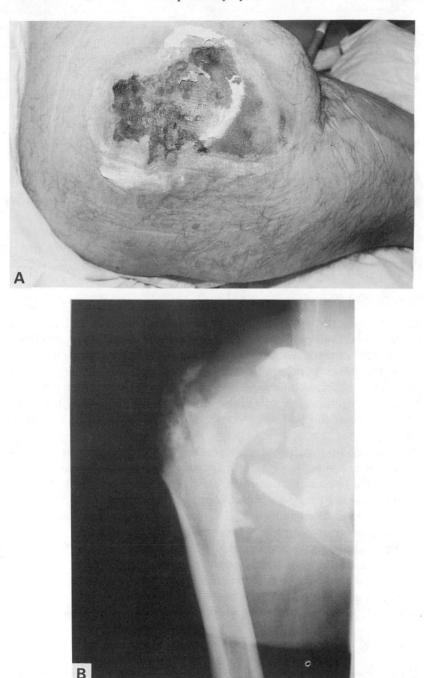

Figure 9.5 Long-standing pressure sore in paraplegic patient. Both the massive new bone formation and destruction of the hip is evident. These complications are seen only in paraplegic patients

patients. It is widespread, particularly obvious around the face and develops only when more than 5 g of protein are lost in the urine per day. However, oedema may well be overlooked, or its significance not appreciated, since many paraplegics suffer from postural oedema of the lower limbs owing to their lack of mobility and prolonged recumbency which impairs the venous return from the lower limbs. A further important cause of oedema in the lower limbs of paraplegic patients is deep venous thrombosis of the lower limbs, which is an almost universal phenomenon.

Haemorrhage

Many patients with amyloidosis suffer from recent small haemorrhages from the mucus membranes, perhaps due to amyloid infiltration of the blood vessels. There are many possible causes of bleeding, such as multiple deficiencies of protein and vitamins and a raised blood pressure and urea due to renal failure.

Toxaemia and Amyloid

Charcot stressed that if pressure sores are infected, they are a source of bacteraemia. Four of the patients from the post-mortem series of Tribe and Silver and 7 of the cases from the Baker *et al.* series died from toxaemia or acute ulcerative endocarditis. They had widespread amyloidosis. The widespread infiltration by amyloid of the bone marrow, lymph glands, gut, liver, spleen and other reticuloendothelial organs impedes the defence mechanisms of the body with consequent susceptibility to overwhelming sepsis.

There was no evidence that amyloidosis prevented pressure sores from healing or interfered with the primary healing of surgical wounds. Many of these patients had severe pressure sores with underlying osteomyelitis, most frequently round the hip. The penetration through to the hip joint was a particularly ominous sign and was associated with toxaemia and a dramatic collapse of the patient.

The treatment of these sores is particularly difficult, since flexor spasms result in movement of the hip with shearing stresses that allow pus to pocket and penetrate around the tissue planes (Figure 9.5). These sores were probably the initial cause of the amyloidosis and the failure to heal was due to local anatomical factors and not to systemic amyloidosis.

Natural History

The natural history of fatal pressure sores is that of large sores that heal and break down involving bone, particularly the femoral head, with persistent sequestra and sinuses. In these patients, death occurs earlier than in other paraplegics, and there is an unusually high incidence of death following acute illness either from sepsis, congestive failure or gastrointes-tinal bleeding, or as a result of infiltration of amyloid into organs as a systemic complication of long-term infection compounded by bony in-volvement. The sores are large, deep and are present for a greater percentage of the patients' lifetime than in other patients. The question as to whether the patients die because of the amyloidosis, or whether it is merely co-existent at death, still remains to be answered. A retrospective study of 65 patients who died with histological evidence of amyloid disease revealed that it developed between 1.5 and 25 years after the paraplegia, with an average survival of 11.8 years (Tribe and Silver, 1969). Many of these cases, however, did not receive adequate treatment by modern standards, some of them having developed paraplegia before special centres were opened. Once the patient has developed amyloidosis, he could lead a fairly healthy life for a few years with very reduced residual renal function as long as severe hypertension is not present. However, once the creatinine clearance falls by 20 ml/min or the serum creatinine rises above 300 mg/ml the prognosis is poor. Complications that can rapidly precipitate a patient with amyloidosis into renal failure or uraemia are episodes of dehydration, haematuria or temporary obstruction of urine flow due to a blocked catheter or a twisted Paul's tubing.

The whole tenor of this chapter illustrates that sores can occur in hospital and that the term applied to paraplegic patients could be changed from pressure and bed sore to hospital sore. A great deal of space has been devoted to showing the injurious factors that prevail in hospital, the defective nursing and the defective use of equipment, malnutrition and toxic factors, but Charcot had very profound thoughts on this very subject, as evidenced by the following observations made over 100 years ago:

There are circumstances in which, contrary to the usual rule, local nutrition may receive a serious blow from the mere fact that a part has been withdrawn from vasomotor innervation. This happens as experiments attest when the whole organism has been subjected to potent debilitating causes, thus a vigorous animal has long had the greater sympathetic nerve divided on the side of the neck: nevertheless, no injury has been experienced in the parts corresponding to the distribution of the divided nerve. But let the animal fall sick or be deprived of food then the scene changes immediately and we see, says M. Claude Bernard, an inflammatory phenomenon ensue in that side of the face which corresponds with the experimental section. On that side, even without the intervention of any external agent whatever, the conjunctiva and pituitary membrane rapidly begin to suppurate. In man, the same concurrence of circumstances ought necessarily to determine effects analogous to those observed in animals. And we may indeed question whether some of our trophic derangements are not really produced in this manner. Such is, perhaps, the case as regards the acute bed sore of apoplectic patients. Here, in fact, the general condition is most unfavourable and the gluteal eschar occupies precisely that side of the body which on account of the motor paralysis presents a relative elevation of temperature evidently connected to the vasomotor hyperaemia. (Charcot, 1877.)

REFERENCES

Baker, J. H. E., Silver, J. R. and Tudway, A. J. C. (1984). Late complications of pressure sores. *Care, Science and Practice*, **3**, 56–59

Breithaupt, D. J., Jousse, A. T. and Wynne-Jones, M. (1961). Late cause of death and life expectancy in paraplegia. *Can. Med. Assoc. J.*, **85**, 73–77

Bright, R. (1821). *Report of Medical Cases*, London, pp. 380–432

Brodie, B. (1836). *Medic. Chirug. Transactions*, 148

Charcot, J.-M. (1877). *On Diseases of the Nervous System*. Translated by Sigerson, G., New Sydenham Society, pp. 63, 126

Cook, J. B. (1961). Scientific aspects of neurology. In Garland, H. (ed.), *Leeds Neurological Sciences Colloquium 1959–60*, Churchill-Livingstone, Edinburgh, Chapter 19, pp. 241–248

Creek, G., Moore, M., Oliver, M., Salisbury, V., Silver, J. R. and Zarb, G. (1987). Personal and social implications of spinal cord injury: A retrospective study. Thames Polytechnic, p. 220

Fabricius, Hildanus (1593). *De gangraena et sphacelo tractatus methodicus*, Leyden

Geisler, W. O., Jousse, A. T. and Wynne-Jones, M. (1977). Survival in traumatic transverse myelitis. *Paraplegia*, **14**, 262–275

Geisler, W. O., Jousse, A. T., Wynne-Jones, M. and Breithaupt, D. J. (1983). Survival in traumatic spinal cord injury. *Paraplegia*, **21**, 364–373

Guttmann, L. (1953). The treatment and rehabilitation of patients with injuries of the spinal cord. In Cope, Z. (ed.), *Medical History of the Second World War, Surgery*. HMSO, London, vol. 2, 422–516

Guttmann, L. (1976). In *Spinal Cord Injuries, Comprehensive Management and Research*. Blackwell Scientific Publications, Oxford, pp. 512–543

Holdsworth, F. (1963). Early orthopaedic treatment of patients with spinal injuries. In Harris, P. (ed.), *Proc. Symp. Spinal Injuries, R. Coll. Surg., Edinburgh*, pp. 93–101 and 160–162

Jousse, A. T., Wynne-Jones, M. and Breithaupt, D. J. (1968). A follow up study of life expectancy and mortality in traumatic transverse myelitis. *Can. Med. Assoc. J.*, **98**, 770–772

Munro, D. (1945). The treatment of patients with injuries of the spinal cord and cauda equina preliminary to making them ambulatory. *Clinics*, **4**, 448–474

Munro, D. (1947). The rehabilitation of patients totally paralysed below the waist with special reference to making them ambulatory and capable of earning their living. III. Tidal drainage, cystometry and bladder training. *New Eng. J. Med.*, **236**, 223–235

Ravichandran, G. and Silver, J. R. (1982). Missed injuries of the spinal cord. *Br. Med. J.*, **284**, 953–960

Richardson, R. R. and Meyer, P. R. (1981). Prevalence and incidence of pressure sores in acute spinal cord injuries. *Paraplegia*, **19**, 235–247

Silver, J. R., Morris, W. R. and Otfinowski, J. S. (1980). Associated injuries in patients with spinal cord injury. *Injury*, **12**, 219–224

Silver, J. R. (1975). Pressure sores, management of complications. Modern Geriatrics, **5**, 6–16

Silver, J. R. and Gibbon, N. O. K. (1968). Prognosis in tetraplegia. *Br. Med. J.*, **4**, 79–83

Silver, J. R., Morris, W. R. and Otfinowski, J. S. (1980). Associated injuries in patients with spinal cord injury. *Injury*, **12**, 219–224

Thompson Walker, J. (1917). Hunterian lecture on the bladder in gunshot and other injuries of the spinal cord. *Lancet*, 173–179

Thompson Walker, J. (1937). The treatment of the bladder in spinal injuries in the war. *Br. J. Urol.*, **9**, 217–230

Thyagarajan, C. and Silver, J. R. (1984). Aetiology of pressure sores in patients with spinal cord injury. *Br. Med. J.*, **289**, 1487–1490

Tribe, C. R. and Silver, J. R. (1969). In *Renal Failure in Praplegia*. Pitman Medical, London, pp. 54–89

10

Reconstructive Surgery

Christopher Khoo and Bruce N. Bailey

INTRODUCTION

The management of pressure sores has always reflected the prevailing beliefs about their cause. Fabricius (1593) held that skin ulceration was caused by a 'pneuma' resulting from loss of nerve and blood supply to the skin. Even Charcot (1868, 1879) believed that pressure ulcers resulted from the action of a neurotrophic factor which caused tissue necrosis. As late as 1940 Munro stated that pressure sores were inevitable following paraplegia, owing to the loss of protective reflexes, and should therefore not be treated.

At the same time however the traditional view was being challenged by Brown-Séquard (1852), whose experimental work showed that cord-injured animals healed as quickly as normal animals and that there was no intrinsic healing deficiency. He believed that pressure sores were due to the deleterious combined effect of pressure and moisture on the skin. In 1861 Florence Nightingale recognised that pressure sores could be prevented when she stated 'if a patient develops a bedsore it is the fault of the nurse and not the fault of the disease'.

Before 1940, a cord-injured patient had an 82 per cent chance of dying within two years. After the Second World War, however, this figure had fallen to 8 per cent (Taylor, 1973) due to the control of urinary and wound infection with antibiotics. After this time it became of great importance to be able to offer adequate treatment to surviving paraplegic patients. The anatomical distribution and incidence of pressure sores have been reviewed by Dansereau and Conway (1964) and are summarised in Table 10.1. Although other studies have shown slightly different relative incidences of pressure sores, the ischial tuberosity, sacrum and greater trochanter remain the most common problem areas.

GENERAL PLAN OF TREATMENT

It is now well accepted that the surgical management of pressure sores almost always includes a number of stages, so that the treatment becomes a

Table 10.1   Anatomical distribution of a series of 1604 pressure sores in 649 patients

Location of ulcer	Number of ulcers	Occurrence (%)
Ischial tuberosity	447	28
Trochanter	310	19
Sacrum	278	17
Heel	138	9
Malleolus	85	5
Pre-tibial area	76	5
Patella	65	4
Other sites	209	13

Based on Dansereau and Conway (1964).

sequential progression through the following stages:

– initial excision of all necrotic and infected tissue from the dirty wound;
– repeated wound excision and dressings to remove every vestige of avascular and infected tissue to achieve a healthy granulating wound; and finally,
– definitive closure of the clean wound. This may be achieved with an initial skin graft, or by primary flap cover.

Initial wound closure is intended to restore the protective skin barrier to prevent continuing protein loss in the wound exudate, and also to prevent infection. The course of hospital treatment is shortened once the wound is closed, and the complications of chronic infection and irritation, such as amyloidosis, osteomyelitis, soft tissue calcification, systemic sepsis and Marjolin's ulcer may be prevented.

The final closure should incorporate removal of any underlying bony prominence, especially in the paraplegic patient, as this would promote the pressure and shearing effects which would predispose to recurrence of the ulcer. The wound should be closed without tension using well-vascularised tissue to provide good soft tissue padding over the bed of the ulcer.

Particular care should be taken to protect the area from pressure until sound tissue healing is established.

THE PROBLEM OF RECURRENCE

The outcome of the surgical closure of a pressure sore closely reflects the primary aetiology. So-called 'acute pressure sores', which occur when elderly patients are bedridden and unable to move following an acute illness, for example, a fractured neck of femur, will often resolve just with dressings and relief of pressure, but over a period of time. Following healing with dressings alone, or by surgical closure, the risk of recurrence is low when the patient returns to the previous normal lifestyle.

However this is not the case with paraplegic patients, as discussed in Chapter 9. Reported recurrence rates in several series have all been high, and earlier hopes that the primary use of large soft-tissue flaps, such as compound musculocutaneous flaps, would provide durable, recurrence-free padding have not been fulfilled.

In planning the course of surgical treatment, the possibility of recurrence should always be borne in mind, as despite patient re-education and careful nursing surveillance there is a high incidence of recurrence in paraplegic patients. The reconstructive surgeon should still be able to offer a secondary procedure to obtain healing after a further breakdown has occurred.

It is therefore essential that the simplest possible procedure which will obtain stable closure should be used at the time of the patient's initial presentation with a pressure sore. When the cellulitis and induration have responded to dressings and debridement, and following bony excision if it is possible at this stage, many pressure sores may be directly closed. There may be instances where a split skin graft will help to close a wound quickly, and the graft may be removed later when the wound margins have softened. This procedure was first reported by Davis in 1938. If no local tissue remains after repeated recurrences, the patient may have to face a radical salvage procedure, such as bilateral upper-thigh amputation with filleting of the thighs for use as large vascularised flaps turned over to resurface the buttock and sacral areas (Chase and White, 1959). This procedure was positively advocated not only for providing the needed tissue, and for reducing body weight and improving mobility, but also for eliminating lower-limb problems such as spasticity, ulceration, and vascular stasis.

THE DEVELOPMENT OF RECONSTRUCTIVE SURGERY

Initial attempts to immediately excise large, infected pressure sores and to drag the wound edges together, often under considerable tension, were uniformly unsuccessful. This led to widespread pessimism among surgeons that healing could be achieved.

Although Marie and Roussy proposed in 1915 that pressure sores occurring in not only debilitated but also paraplegic patients could be both prevented and treated, it was only in 1945 that Lamon and Alexander reported Scoville's success the previous year in achieving surgical closure of a sacral sore, using penicillin cover. Further successful procedures were reported by White and Hamm (1946), and in 1947 Conway and others described a variety of procedures for the surgical management of pressure sores, including rotation flaps, skin grafts and Z-plasties.

Also in 1947, Kostrubala and Greeley first stressed the importance of excision of bony prominences to allow wound closure without tension, and also to prevent local recurrence of pressure. Griffith and Schultz (1961) reviewed a series of 1000 cases and found that simple wound excision of trochanteric sores, including superficial bone removal, resulted in 83 per cent healing with a recurrence rate of 20 per cent, while radical bone excision and flap cover resulted in 92 per cent healing with a 6 per cent recurrence rate. In the same series, a recurrence rate of 54 per cent following closure of ischial sores was reduced to 22 per cent if the ischium was totally excised.

In 1948 Bors and Comarr suggested that muscle transposed into a pressure sore defect might help to diffuse pressure, and reported use of the gluteus maximus muscle as a rotation flap. However, muscle is more susceptible to the effects of pressure-induced ischaemia than skin (Keane, 1978), and experimental studies in a rat model have shown that even when the overlying skin appears normal the muscle component of a musculocutaneous flap atrophies. Clinically this leads to loss of the original thick layer of muscle, which becomes replaced by a thinner sheet of fibrous scar. The biological function of muscle is to contract, not to bear weight.

The anatomical basis for vascularised flaps was not properly understood when such flaps were first used on an empirical basis. It had been found that many compound flaps containing muscle and all overlying sub-cutaneous tissue and skin could be successfully transposed and would completely survive (Bailey, 1967). However, such flap transfers were based on individual surgeons' experiences of previous flap survival rather than the knowledge of a predictable pattern of blood supply.

In 1972, McGregor and Jackson defined the vascular basis of the groin flap, which depended on a specific pattern of cutaneous arteries for survival. The concept of such 'axial' flaps, which could be designed to include and be extended along the course of specific arteries, has become of crucial importance in reconstructive surgery.

Other such axial flaps relevant to pressure sore reconstruction make use of arteries supplying specific muscles, and which ramify to the overlying skin, such as the original Tensor Fascia Lata musculocutaneous flap of Bailey, and developed by Nahai and colleagues (1978, 1979). These may be designed as muscle, or skin and muscle (musculocutaneous) flaps. The indications for particular flaps are discussed below in relation to specific pressure sore defects. It should be remembered that the muscle portion of a musculocutaneous flap may provide initial padding, but its main function is to act as a carrier for blood supply, which reaches the skin through the muscle. The muscle loses its physiological function as a contractile tissue.

As an extension of this concept it has been possible to take large flaps of vascularised tissue from distant sites, for immediate transfer to distant pressure sore defects, with immediate reconnection of the axial artery and vein using microsurgical techniques. This procedure has been described for the reconstruction of large sacral defects using a single filleted lower leg musculocutaneous free flap from an amputated limb (Chen *et al.*, 1986).

The tensor fascia lata flap is innervated by the lateral cutaneous branch of the iliohypogastric nerve (T_{12}) and the lateral femoral cutaneous nerve (L_2 and L_3) and may allow sensate reconstruction in some paraplegic patients (Cochran *et al.*, 1981). Attempts have also been made to re-innervate flaps to restore sensation to the area of the pressure sore by using long nerve grafts to restore sensation from above the level of the cord injury (Daniel *et al.*, 1976). These techniques have not been universally successful in achieving and maintaining healing through restoration of sensation.

It is open to discussion whether extensive flap techniques should be used primarily. While large musculocutaneous flaps provide good soft-tissue padding, they do not necessarily prevent the recurrences of ulceration which are extremely common in paraplegic patients. Recent series have clearly shown that the incidence of recurrence is higher in patients in whom large musculocutaneous flaps have been used primarily (Palmer, 1987), possibly because reconstruction was not followed by the essential preventive measures when the patients were discharged. There is also the major problem that secondary reconstruction of ulceration occurring in the same site is difficult if the needed tissue was already used in the initial surgical procedure.

Goals of Surgical Management

Successful closure of the pressure sore achieves benefits through:

1. Prevention of local and systemic infection.
2. Prevention of protein loss and catabolism.
3. Avoidance of long-term complications, e.g. amyloidosis, renal failure, malignant change.
4. Improved patient management, including hygiene and comfort.
5. Reduction in duration and cost of hospital care.

PRINCIPLES OF FLAP DESIGN

While specific anatomical details are of course different in each site, the principles of treatment remain the same for each area and their application in each site will be discussed in detail below.

Table 10.2 Classification of flaps used in surgical reconstruction of pressure sore defects

Geometrical design
Advancement
Rotation
  with back-cut
  with out-cut
Transposition

Anatomical content
Cutaneous
Fascio-cutaneous
Muscle
Musculocutaneous

Blood supply
Random cutaneous
Axial (arterial)
  pedicled
  free (microsurgical)

The flaps used for the reconstruction of pressure sore defects are segments of perfused tissue which are designed, dissected and moved in order to fit into a defect which could not otherwise be closed. They may contain skin and fascia, or may also include an underlying muscle in order to take advantage of its intrinsic blood supply which will adequately nourish the overlying skin. Flaps can therefore be classified by their tissue content as detailed in Table 10.2.

It is also basic to flap design that, wherever possible, the flap should contain a known artery or arteries in its pedicle, which will reliably perfuse the tissue contained in the flap. The principle of 'axial' or arterial flaps has been alluded to above and is shown in Figure 10.1.

Flaps may also be described in terms of their geometrical design. Thus the tissue may be advanced, or dissected free enough to be pulled into the defect under acceptable tension (advancement flap), or be rotated around the circumference of a circle (rotation flap), or swung like a pendulum to fit an adjacent defect (transposition flap) (Figure 10.2). The movement of the flap tissue always creates a secondary defect. Small secondary defects may be closed directly by undermining and advancement of adjacent skin margins, but skin grafts may be needed to close large defects. These areas are planned to lie over a smooth, well-muscled surface where the presence of a skin graft will not create difficulties, or prevent the patient from taking weight.

Following an adequate bone excision, when closure by simpler methods is not possible, it may be useful to consider the transposition of a muscle flap. A number of muscles, such as the gracilis in the thigh, or the gastrocnemius in the lower leg, have an independent blood supply running

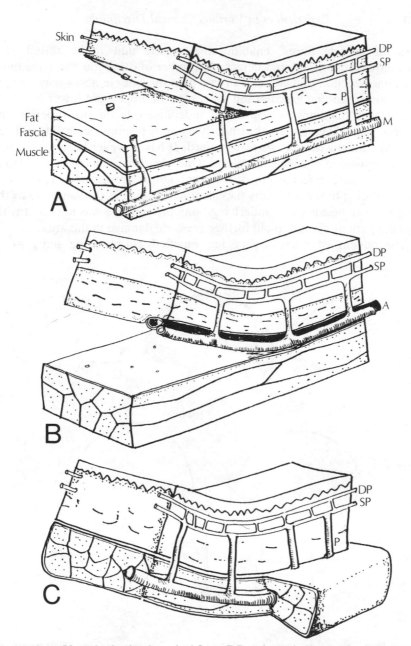

Figure 10.1 Vascular basis of surgical flaps. DP = dermal plexus, SP = subdermal plexus, P = musculocutaneous perforating artery; A = axial skin artery and vein; M = muscular artery. (A) 'Random' pattern skin flap, dependent on intrinsic skin vessels within dermal and subdermal vascular plexi. (B) Axial, or arterial, flap incorporating defined cutaneous artery and venae comitantes. (C) Musculocutaneous flap, in which a defined muscular artery supplies the overlying skin through perforating arteries. Large amounts of overlying skin are supplied and large flaps may be raised for pressure sore reconstruction with excellent viability

into the muscle fibres, enabling the muscle unit to be raised as a vascularised flap to fill in a defect. A number of other muscles have more than one vascular pedicle, and in this case the muscle fibres may be split into more than one vascularised unit, e.g. the upper and lower halves of the gluteus maximus muscle based independently on the superior and inferior gluteal vessels. As the underlying bony prominence will have been excised, the muscle may be skin-grafted. It has however been shown that the transposition of a well-vascularised muscle or musculocutaneous flap to a pressure sore defect is not of itself enough to prevent recurrence. It is disappointing to see a healthy flap ulcerate through in the same site as the original sore because the underlying bony prominence was not dealt with, and the patient did not avoid further pressure damage in the area.

The advent of microsurgery has enabled entire tissue units to be

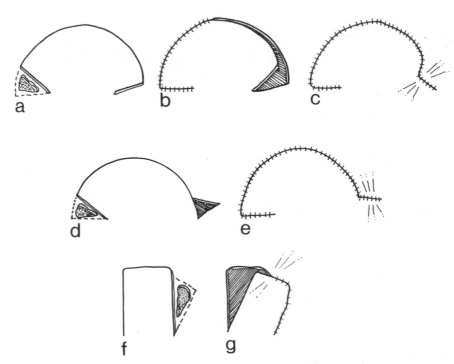

Figure 10.2 Geometrical design of skin flaps: (a–e) rotation flaps, (f, g) transposition flap. (a) Defect triangulated, and rotation flap designed with a 'back-cut' into the base. (b) Flap rotated to close defect, leaving secondary defect, which may be closed directly, (c). (d) Alternatively the flap may be designed with an 'out-cut', and direct closure may be achieved (e). The choice of design should take into account the availability of tissue for closure of the secondary defect. (f, g) Diagrammatic representation of closure of defect with a transposition flap. The secondary defect (seen in (g)) will usually require a skin graft for closure

completely severed from their donor sites and transposed to different areas of the body. Perfusion is immediately restored by suture of the artery and vein to suitable vessels in the recipient site. Attempts have also been made to re-innervate these transferred flaps, by connecting them via long nerve grafts to sensory nerves arising from above the level of the neurological injury.

SURGICAL MANAGEMENT

Before the patient can be successfully operated upon, three basic conditions must be satisfied, as follows.

Relief of Pressure on the Wound

The patient must be nursed in a position which allows complete relief of pressure on the ulcerated area. However, care must be taken to ensure that other areas which might be at risk are adequately protected.

The common sites of pressure ulceration, i.e. the ischium, sacrum, and trochanter, are all protected when the patient is lying prone. The *anterior* pressure areas, the anterior iliac spines, knees, etc., must be safeguarded. This position allows access for dressings, and is facilitated by movable pillows and packs, or by sophisticated beds which use inflated low-air-loss sacs or fluidised beads to achieve even distribution of weight.

If the patient is to be nursed in the lateral position, it is important that regular turns are instituted so that no area at risk is subjected to pressure for a prolonged period. Unfortunately, it is not uncommon for patients who are being treated for sacral pressure sores, for example, to develop secondary trochanteric pressure sores because they are left for too long on their sides.

Wound Management

All infected and necrotic tissue should be excised. This is readily done at the bedside at the time of regular wound dressings. In the first instance, access may be improved to a large undermined cavity by incising and laying open the cavity, under local anaesthesia if necessary. The necrotic tissue is excised by scalpel or scissor dissection, and if the dissection is confined to necrotic tissue, there is no reason why the patient should suffer discomfort even if the area is sensate. Thick, blackened eschars may be excised by deep scoring and softening with regular applications of 0.2 per cent nitrofurazone cream, followed by serial excision.

The wound is packed with antiseptic-soaked gauze, and in the initial stages when there is heavy contamination, sodium hypochlorite (Eusol) or aqueous povidone iodine dressings are appropriate. The packing gauze is wrung out so that it is barely moist. As it dries further, the surface slough adheres to the gauze and is pulled out as the pack is changed. At a later stage when the wound is clean, the moistening agent may be changed to a solution such as sterile saline which does not inhibit the formation of granulation tissue. It may be necessary to repeat the dressings two to three times a day in the initial stages when there is marked infection.

The excised tissue may be sent for quantitative bacterial culture, and it is important to be aware that surface wound swabs may not reflect the extent of bacterial colonisation. Wound healing does not occur until the bacterial count is less than 10^5 organisms per gram of tissue. It is important to request anaerobic cultures: gram-negative faecal organisms are common pathogens in the sacral, ischial and trochanteric areas.

Antibiotics are *contra-indicated* at this stage: the ulcers will be surrounded by fibrosis through which adequate penetration may not be possible. Thus the minimal inhibitory concentration will not be reached in the tissue of the ulcer itself and there may be the development of bacterial resistance. Antibiotics should be given if there are signs of systemic sepsis, and should be specifically targeted, on the basis of bacterial isolates during the wound dressing phase, to cover the period of surgical reconstruction.

The goal of pre-operative wound care is to produce a clean ulcer, without visible necrotic tissue, lined by vascular granulation tissue which is dry, bright in appearance, and without an offensive odour. At the same time the wound margins will have begun to contract and a fine fringe of healthy new epithelium will be visible. At this stage the wound is in a position to heal spontaneously with continued care. Surgical intervention is therefore held back until such time as the wound has entered a favourable healing phase.

Assessment and Care of the Patient

Wound dressings, pressure avoidance, and the control of infection are specific measures directed at the pressure sore, but it is also important not to lose sight of the needs of the patient as a whole.

Nutrition

Many patients with longstanding pressure sores will be markedly catabolic. The effects of the acute illness which predisposed to the development of pressure ulceration will have been compounded by chronic protein loss from the wound, and by the inevitable secondary infection.

Table 10.3 Basic nutritional requirements of patients with pressure sores

CALORIES	3000–6000 kcal/24 h	
PROTEIN	2–3 × normal requirement	
VITAMINS	A, B complex, C	
TRACE ELEMENTS		
	zinc	660 mg/24 h
	magnesium	350 mg/24 h
	calcium	0.8–1.2 g/24 h
	copper	0.5–2.0 mg/24 h

Table 10.4 Nutritional assessment of patients with pressure sores

Clinical assessment
– 24-hour urine collection
– serum albumin ([a]more than 35 g/l)
– serum transferrin ([a]more than 2 g/l)
– body weight

Biochemical assessment
Calculation of protein catabolised

$$\frac{\text{urine urea (mmol)}}{5} = \text{protein catabolised/24 h (g)}$$

Derivation of calculation

daily urine urea loss	$[u]$ mmol/24 h
60 g urea = 1 mol : 1 mmol =	60/1000
proportion of urinary N_2 loss	6/5
N_2 : urea molecular weight ratio	28/60
1 g nitrogen =	6.25 g protein

$$\text{protein loss} = [u] \times \frac{60}{1000} \times \frac{28}{60} \times \frac{6}{5} \times 6.25$$

or $\quad\dfrac{[u]}{5}$ approximately

[a]Desirable levels.

Early wound closure will help to control the hypercatabolic state. Initial closure with a simple temporary technique is often advisable, even if it is intended to follow with definitive reconstruction using a more robust flap. Subsequent surgery will then be carried out in a fitter patient who is better able to tolerate more extensive surgery and to heal uneventfully.

The ordinary ward diet is inadequate. The daily nutritional requirement in a pressure sore patient is likely to be several times greater than the normal basal requirement, as listed in Table 10.3. The patient's dietary intake should be assessed: a formal nitrogen balance is useful, but simple measures such as a weekly body weight, serum albumin, and 24-hour urine urea excretion should be monitored. The table also includes a useful calculation of protein catabolism. Additional vitamin and trace element supplements should also be considered. If the patient is anorexic, or unable for any reason to take an adequate diet by mouth, fine-bore nasogastric tube feeding, a feeding gastrostomy, or short-term intravenous hyperalimentation should be considered. These techniques are not distressing to the patient. Continuous intravenous infusion, or continuous pumped tube feeding may be the only means of giving patients an adequate protein and calorie intake to render them fit for surgery.

Anaemia

Blood loss can be significant, especially during the pre-operative stage when frequent wound debridements are being carried out to prepare the wound for surgery. There is also further blood loss during and after the operation, especially when bone is excised, or large soft-tissue flaps are raised for reconstruction. There may also be further bleeding from skin graft donor sites.

It is desirable that the patient's haemoglobin level should be maintained at 10 g/dl or more. At this relatively low level there is in fact an ideal balance between low blood viscosity and adequate oxygen transport, so that perfusion of tissue flaps is satisfactorily maintained.

The need for blood transfusion should be monitored with regular blood counts, and any specific abnormalities seen on the blood film should be investigated and treated, e.g. macrocytosis, or hypochromasia.

Paraplegic Patients

Concurrent problems associated with paraplegic patients with pressure sores must also be managed. They have been discussed in detail in Chapter 9.

PRESSURE SORES IN SPECIFIC SITES

The Ischial Tuberosity

Anatomical features

The ischial tuberosity is the bony prominence at the angular junction of the vertically running ischial body, and the transversely disposed ischial ramus. It gives rise to a number of muscles, including some fibres of adductor magnus, as well as the inferior gemellus and quadratus femoris. None of these muscles is indispensable.

The fascia overlying the tuberosity is loculated into compartments by intersecting fibrous septa, which help to form a cushion-like layer of fat and fibrous tissue.

Although this bony prominence is covered by the gluteus maximus muscle in the erect posture, these muscle fibres slide out of the way in the sitting posture so that weight is taken directly over the bony prominence. This is well illustrated in Figures 14.1 and 14.2. The bony tuberosity is often covered by an anatomical bursa lying between the tuberosity and the posterior margin of gluteus maximus: minor degrees of pressure-induced inflammation are well known, the condition being known as 'tailor's bottom' or 'weaver's bottom'.

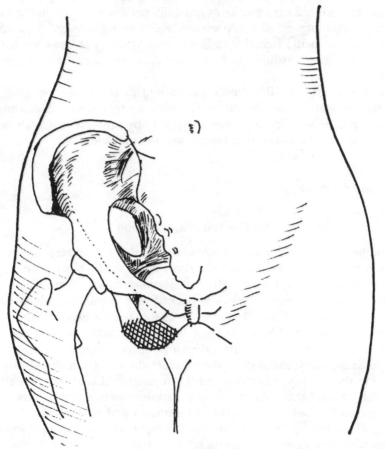

Figure 10.3 Ischial pressure sores: anatomy. The cross-hatched area of ischial tuberosity is resected when the overlying pressure sore and bursa are removed

Pathology

When pressure-induced ulceration occurs, the bursa becomes infected, and the infection extends from the prominence of the ischial tuberosity below (Figure 10.3) through to the overlying skin. There is associated fat necrosis, and depending on the patient's posture, the infection may extend laterally into the hip joint, or into the groin or the posterior thigh.

The small surface opening into the pressure sore may well belie the extensive cavity beneath, the true extent of which may be shown by the injection of radio-opaque contrast into the cavity.

Conservative Management

Many acute ischial sores, if not most, will heal spontaneously in response to adequate wound care measures once the patient is placed in the prone position, avoiding all direct pressure over the tuberosity. A common situation is the acute ischial sore in the patient who has been left for too long in a sitting posture: bedrest and dressings alone are extremely effective.

As in the case of all patients put to bed in the prone position, the anterior pressure areas should be carefully protected so that secondary ulceration does not develop over anterior bony prominences such as the ribs, the anterior superior iliac spines, and the patellae.

Surgical Treatment

Wound and Bone Excision

When the wound is clean and in a favourable state for surgery, the patient is treated by en-bloc excision of the sore, down to the bony prominence. This is most easily achieved with the 'pseudotumour' technique (Figure 10.4) in which the wound cavity is packed with povidone iodine-soaked gauze, firmly stitched into the cavity to enable total excision of the entire cavity in one mass. The underlying bony prominence is then exposed. There is controversy about the extent of bone excision needed: while a full-thickness bony excision is undoubtedly the most effective means of reducing the bony prominence, many surgeons feel that this procedure, especially when carried out bilaterally, exposes the perineal soft tissues to pressure so that secondary perineal ulceration and urethral fistulae may occur. This complication has long been recognised, and was seen in up to 58 per cent of patients undergoing bilateral radical ischiectomy (Bors and Comarr, 1958), and has recently been the subject of careful pressure studies (Hackler and Zampieri, 1987).

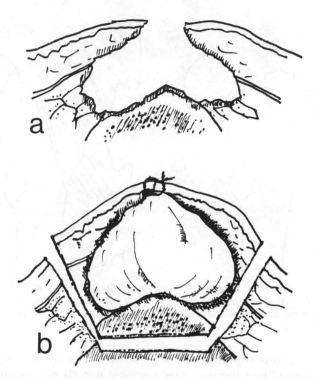

Figure 10.4 'Pseudotumour' technique for pressure sore excision. (a) The wound extends deeply to the underlying bony prominence. Periostitis and osteomyelitis may be present. (b) An iodine-soaked pack is sutured into the cavity, and the ulcer and bone are resected *en bloc*

Adequate exposure is obtained through a sub-periosteal approach, using an elevator to strip the soft tissues and periosteum from the symphysis medially to the obturator externus laterally. The bone projection may be markedly reduced using precision cuts from an air-powered osteotome, or powered saw. Full-thickness excision may be accomplished by hand with a Gigli saw, or using powered instruments.

Wound Closure

Following the removal of the ulcer and the ischial tuberosity, it is almost always possible to achieve direct soft tissue closure. The exception to this is when there has been longstanding infection with a marked degree of secondary scarring which has caused extensive induration, so preventing the skin edges from closing together.

It is emphasised that the solitary ischial sore is almost always amenable to direct closure. Exceptionally flap closure may be helpful. The inferior

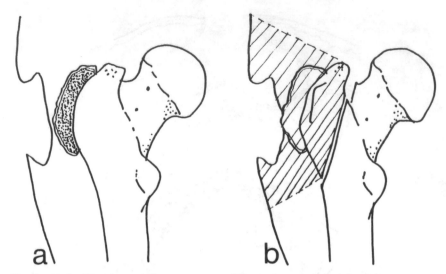

Figure 10.5   Excision of the greater trochanter for trochanteric pressure sores. The bursa underlying the sore may be extensively infected. *En-bloc* excision should include the entire area of the ulcer, the bursa, and the bony prominence of the greater trochanter

half of the gluteus maximus muscle may be raised on the inferior gluteal vessels and turned into the defect as a muscle flap. If skin closure is not possible a skin graft may be applied. Gracilis muscle or musculocutaneous flaps will also effectively close the defect of an ischial sore. The tensor fascia lata musculocutaneous flap is particularly useful for the closure of multiple adjacent sores, such as coexisting ischial and trochanteric sores (Figure 10.5).

A large gluteal rotation flap may be designed to include the gluteal fascia, with its circumference planned to lie below the prominence of the iliac crest so that the margin of the flap will not lie over the bony prominence. Laterally, the margin passes over the trochanteric area, and towards the ischium. A large flap will allow closure with least tension, and can be raised again and further rotated or transposed to serve for cover should a further breakdown occur. Movement of the flap leaves a secondary defect which may be closed by excising a triangle at the base of the flap, or by back-cutting inwards into the base.

Trochanteric Sores

Anatomical Features

The bony mass of the greater trochanter gives rise to the vastus lateralis muscle, and provides a strong insertion for the gluteal muscles. There is little soft-tissue padding over the bony prominence, and ulceration may progress to a deeply undermined cavity with secondary osteomyelitis.

Surgical Treatment

Bone Excision

Radical excision of the greater trochanter should be included in any surgical treatment of pressure sores in this area. If the condition is longstanding and has developed sinuses extending deeply into bone it is also necessary to excise the entire neck of femur and even part of the acetabulum, to fully eliminate infection. A muscle flap may then be necessary to obliterate the resulting dead space.

The greater trochanter may be excised by serial osteotome cuts passing smoothly from the trochanteric fossa to the upper outer aspect of the femoral shaft (Figure 10.6). It may be possible to obtain deep closure with periosteal flaps, but if there has been infection the periosteum will be of poor quality. The bleeding cancellous bone surface may be sealed with bovine collagen paste. However, bone wax may act as a focus for infection and should not be used.

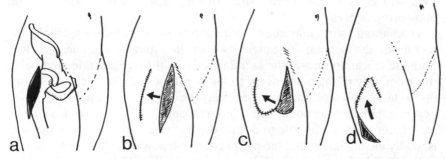

Figure 10.6 Some skin flaps for closure of throchanteric defects. (a) Direct closure may be possible. (b) Closure with a bipedicled flap. (c) Superiorly based transposition flap. This may be designed as a musculocutaneous flap to include the tensor fascia lata muscle. (d) Anteriorly based transposition flap. Note that (b), (c) and (d) require a skin graft for closure of the secondary defect

Wound Closure

There is ample local tissue for closure, which can often be achieved by simple advancement of the skin margins when the defect is less than 40 mm in width. Random skin flaps may be based superiorly or anteriorly and

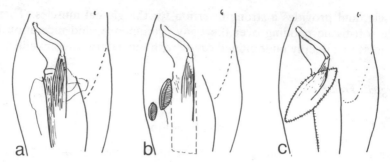

Figure 10.7 Tensor fascia lata musculocutaneous flap. (a) The muscle arises from the anterior superior iliac crest and the notch between the superior and inferior iliac spines. Its anterior border is easily defined and forms the anterior border of the skin territory, (b). A very long superiorly based flap may be transposed to resurface both trochanteric and ischial sores in continuity, or the flap may be incised all round ('island flap', (c)) to allow closure without a contour irregularity or 'dog ear.' The donor site may often be closed directly as in (c). The transposition flap design is preferred if it is intended to preserve innervation from the lateral cutaneous branch of the iliohypogastric nerve (T_{12}), which enters the flap from above and posteriorly, or the lateral femoral cutaneous nerve (L_2, L_3), which enters from above and anteriorly

transposed to provide good cover, with the secondary defect being covered by a skin graft on the lateral aspect of the thigh, a smooth area without bony prominences.

Trochanteric sores may coexist with ulceration in other sites, chiefly the sacrum or the ischium. A gluteal rotation flap may be designed to close both the trochanteric and the sacral sore, with the trochanteric area being the secondary triangle necessary to allow rotation of the flap. The tensor fascia lata musculocutaneous flap may be used as a superiorly based pedicled flap, and the donor site is often amenable to direct closure. It may be geometrically preferable to design the flap as an 'island' where the skin is totally incised all around the margin of the flap, which remains connected only through its muscular and vascular pedicle (Figure 10.7). Other island flaps from the thigh may be used, such as the biceps femoris flap in which a paddle of skin is transported on a vascularised muscle pedicle. The secondary defect can usually be closed directly.

Sacral Sores

Anatomical Features

The five sacral vertebrae form a bony prominence which is convex posteriorly. The median sacral crest is formed by the spinous processes, and is thronged either side by the posterior sacral foramina. A further bony ridge, the lateral sacral crest, lies lateral to the foramina on each side and in thin patients both of these bony ridges may give rise to pressure, as may the sacral tuberosities and the posterior superior spines of the iliac crests. When infection occurs, the fibres of the supraspinous, sacrococcygeal, and sacroiliac ligaments may become involved. In patients with extensive ischial and sacral sores, the infection may spread along a plane above the sacrotuberous ligaments to create a large undermined cavity which is more extensive than the ulcer in the overlying skin.

The gluteus maximus muscles arise on each side from the posterior gluteal line of the ilium, and towards the mid-line from the sacrotuberous ligaments. This muscle has a versatile role in reconstructive surgery in the sacral area, and may be detached from its origin and advanced medially, or incorporated in the design of musculocutaneous flaps which take advantage of two separate vascular pedicles which supply the superior and inferior halves of the gluteus maximus. Thus the upper and lower halves of each muscle may be split into independent vascular units, and the muscle flaps may be based superiorly and turned over into the sacral defect, or inferiorly as part of a musculocutaneous rotation flap.

Surgical Treatment

Bone Excision

There is a basic distinction between the 'acute' sacral pressure sore, which occurs in the sensate patient during the course of an acute illness when the patient is put to bed, and the 'chronic' sacral sore which occurs in the insensate patient with paraplegia or a neurological lesion. Acute pressure sores in the sacral area will usually heal spontaneously with dressings alone, but longstanding sores should be treated as in every other case of chronic pressure ulceration with infection, by excision of the bony prominences to leave an underlying plane surface which will not present a residual bony projection.

Except in paraplegic patients or those with neurological lesions, the avoidance of nerve damage should be constantly borne in mind. Dissection should not pass anterior to the sacrum as there may be troublesome bleeding from the sacral venous plexus, and the median and lateral sacral arteries.

Unfortunately it is not uncommon to see recurrent ulceration occurring through the fresh skin graft or flap used to cover a previous sacral ulcer because bone resection has been neglected. A power osteotome will allow smooth and easily controlled bone resection. In thin paraplegic patients with a prominent coccyx, the coccyx may either be excised or fractured at the sacrococcygeal joint and displaced anteriorly with firm pressure.

Wound Closure

If there is adequate local soft tissue, a clean sacral sore will progressively cicatrise, contracting the defect in size and leaving a stable scar. Wound closure may be achieved by excision and direct suture. If the buttock tissues are tight, many acute sacral sores will still heal spontaneously by epithelialisation, when the granulations will be covered by a layer of fresh, but thin epithelium. This is however poorly resistant to trauma and it may be preferable to achieve permanent cover with a thicker, padded flap.

Rotation flaps for sacral sore closure may be designed to include skin and fascia, or the underlying gluteus maximus muscles as well (Figure 10.8). The inferiorly based design allows a comfortable rotation to close the sacral defect: very large defects may require the use of bilateral flaps. Many variants have been described: the medial attachments of the gluteus maximus may be detached and both musculocutaneous flaps advanced medially to meet in the mid-line, or parts of the muscle may be turned over as a vascularised unit and skin grafted. Many other surgical possibilities have been described, but many should be critically rejected because their design accepts the presence of scars in a weight-bearing area, or the use of skin grafts instead of more robust local flaps.

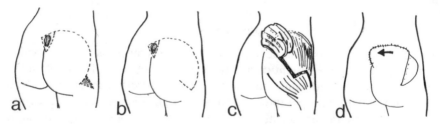

Figure 10.8 Flaps for sacral closure   (a) Inferiorly based rotation flap with 'out-cut', and (b) inferiorly based rotation flap with back-cut. (c) Gluteus maximus muscle flap. The upper half of the muscle may be split from the lower half as it has an independent blood supply. The muscle is turned over to fill the sacral defect, where it is covered by a skin graft. (d) Re-use of a rotation flap. Should recurrent ulceration occur, the previous rotation flap may be raised again and transposed to fill the new defect. A skin graft will then be necessary to close the secondary defect

Other Areas

The principles discussed above for the care and reconstruction of the three commonest areas of pressure ulceration may successfully be applied to other anatomical sites where ulceration also occurs over bony prominences. The approach and practical details are the same: wound debridement is followed by surgical closure using the simplest possible technique. Bone excision may be necessary and should be adequate to eliminate bony pressure points. Specific details of treatment procedures have been described elsewhere (Bailey and Khoo, 1986).

POST-OPERATIVE MANAGEMENT

The closed wounds should be managed with vacuum drainage to prevent the collection of blood or serous exudate which may become infected. A layered closure is preferred, using monofilament, slowly absorbable sutures, which continue to support the wound edges until strong healing is present. Removable external sutures may be necessary, but will create permanent suture marks if left in for long periods, while some loss of strength may occur if the sutures are removed early, within the first few weeks. Additional external support with skin tapes is helpful.

It is particularly imporant to avoid pressure on the skin and soft tissue brought into the area during the surgical reconstruction. Indeed, fresh tissue flaps are particularly vulnerable to the effects of ischaemia which might occur if the patient were allowed to lie on the reconstructed sore immediately. Capillary perfusion pressure is reduced even when special low-air-loss or fluidised bead beds are in use, and if possible pressure should still be avoided for the first few days after the operation.

The patient is allowed to start to take weight on the area when it is soundly healed: initially only for short periods, and under nursing surveillance, and with proper use of pressure-diffusing devices such as cushions, fleeces and conforming bases. Even so it is still important that pressure should be relieved by the patient performing 'lifts' off the weight-bearing areas so as to allow periodic perfusion of the healed area and the new soft-tissue cover. Paraplegic and other neurologically compromised patients must understand that successful healing is not a permanent guarantee against recurrent ulceration. They must themselves be prepared to be vigilant and accept responsibility for care of their own pressure areas and the continuing avoidance of pressure.

REFERENCES

Bailey, B. N. (1967). In *Bedsores*, Edward Arnold, London, pp. 88–89
Bailey, B. N. and Khoo, C. T. K. (1986). In Barclay, T. L. and Kernahan, D. A. (eds), *Rob and Smith's Operative Surgery*, Butterworths, London, pp. 696–712
Bors, E. and Comarr, E. (1948). Ischial decubitus ulcer. *Surgery*, **24**, 680–694
Bors, E. and Comarr, E. (1958). Perineal urethral diverticulum: complication of removal of the ischium. *Journal of the American Medical Association*, **168**, 2000–2003
Brown-Sequard, E. (1852). Experimental researches applied to physiology and pathology. *Med. Exam.*, **8**, 481–504

Charcot, J. M. (1868). In *Arch. Physiol. norm. et Pathol.*, Paris, **1**, 308

Charcot, J. M. (1879). In *Lectures on Diseases of the Nervous System*, 2nd edn, translated by G. Sigerson, Henry C. Lea, Philadelphia

Chase, R. A. and White, W. L. (1959). Bilateral amputation in rehabilitation of paraplegics. *Plastic & Reconstructive Surgery*, **24**, 445–455

Chen, H., Weng, C. and Noordhoff, M. S. (1986). Coverage of multiple extensive pressure sores with a single filleted lower leg myocutaneous free flap. *Plastic and Reconstructive Surgery*, **78**, 396–398

Cochran, J. H., Jr, Edstrom, L. E. and Dibell, D. G. (1981). Usefulness of the innervated tensor fascia lata flap in paraplegic patients. *Annals of Plastic Surgery*, **7**, 286–288

Conway, H., Kraissl, C. J. and Clifford, R. H. (1947). The plastic surgical closure of decubitus ulcers in patients with paraplegia. *Surgery, Gynecology & Obstetrics*, **85**, 321–332

Daniel, R. K., Terzis, J. K. and Cunningham, D. M. (1976). Sensory skin flaps for coverage of pressure sores in paraplegic patients: a preliminary report. *Plastic and Reconstructive Surgery*, **58**, 317–328

Dansereau, J. G. and Conway, H. (1964). Closure of decubiti in paraplegic patients. *Plastic and Reconstructive Surgery*, **33**, 474–480

Davis, J. S. (1938). The operative treatment of scars following bedsores. *Surgery*, **3**, 1–7

Fabricius, Hildanus (1593). In *De gangraena et sphacelo tractatus methodicus*, Leyden

Griffith, B. H. and Schultz, R. C. (1961). The prevention and surgical treatment of recurrent decubitus ulcers in patients with paraplegia. *Plastic & Reconstructive Surgery*, **27**, 248–260

Hackler, R. H. and Zampieri, T. A. (1987). Urethral complications following ischiectomy in spinal cord injury patients: a urethral pressure study. *Journal of Urology*, **137**, 253–255

Keane, F. X. (1978). The function of the rump in relation to sitting and the Keane reciprocating wheelchair seat. *Paraplegia*, **16**, 390–402

Kostrubala, J. G. and Greeley, P. W. (1947). The problem of decubitus ulcers in paraplegics. *Plastic & Reconstructive Surgery*, **2**, 403–412

Lamon, J. D., Jr and Alexander, E., Jr (1945). Secondary closure of decubitus ulcers with the aid of penicillin. *Journal of the American Medical Association*, **127**, 396

McGregor, I. A. and Jackson, I. T. (1972). The groin flap. *British Journal of Plastic Surgery*, **25**, 3–16

Marie, P. and Roussy, G. (1915). *Bull. Société Méd. de Paris*, **73**, 602

Munro, D. (1940). Care of the back following spinal cord injuries: a consideration of bedsores. *New England Medical Journal*, **223**, 391–398

Nahai, F., Silverston, J. S. and Hill, H. L. (1978). The tensor fascia lata musculocutaneous flap. *Annals of Plastic Surgery*, **1**, 372–379

Nahai, F., Hill, H. L. and Hester, T. R. (1979). Experiences with the tensor fascia lata flap. *Plastic and Reconstructive Surgery*, **63**, 788–799

Nightingale, Florence (1861). In *Notes on Nursing*, Appleton Century, New York

Palmer, B. (1987). *Pressure Sores: Prevention of Recurrence*. Paper given at IX Meeting, International Society for Plastic and Reconstructive Surgery, New Delhi

Taylor, R. (1973). Spinal cord injury: its many complications. *American Family Physician*, **8**, 138–146

White, J. C. and Hamm, W. G. (1946). Primary closure of bedsores by plastic surgery. *Annals of Surgery*, **124**, 1136–1147

Part III
Scientific Aspects of Pressure Sores

11

Cellular Responses to Tissue Distortion

Terence J. Ryan

INTRODUCTION

In this chapter the role of mechanical forces in the transduction of biochemical signals will be discussed. Most cells or tissues subjected to mechanical forces resist distortion because any strain is taken by stable and inflexible fibrillar or skeletal elements. Actin, collagen, elastin and fibrin are examples of skeletal proteins. In certain circumstances these skeletal proteins can be lysed by proteases and it is therefore important to protect them from such lysis if the skeleton is to be maintained. In a discussion of how the skin may protect itself against mechanical forces, it was conceived that inhibitors of proteases are synthesised in response to forces tending to distort (Ryan, 1985, 1988). Unfortunately, such inhibitors are not always of benefit. Clots, scars and corns are examples of a failure of the subtle balances in moulding and remoulding that may depend on protease activation and inhibition. It may be simplistic to assume that the only important consequence of pressure or shearing forces on the skin is hypoxia, due to impairment of blood flow. It could be that susceptibility to sores or failure in healing of such is affected by subtle imbalances in the biochemical signals transduced by mechanical forces. Design faults in skeletal tissue, and alterations in the anatomical configuration of skeletal proteins as a consequence of wounding or ageing, may account for special vulnerability or increased susceptibility to decubitus ulceration.

Gravitational Forces

Gravitational forces which account for the effects of weight on the obliteration of blood supply over bony points are also blamed for the susceptibility of the leg to ulceration from venous hypertension. Most physicians rely on concepts of hypoxia to explain such an effect, but the importance of hydrostatic or oncotic pressure has been under-estimated. Even the normal healthy lower leg differs from the upper arm in the distensibility of the tissue (Mridha and Odman, 1985), almost certainly owing to a response to gravitationally induced tissue fluids, which contribute to the inertial elastic and frictional properties of tissues.

The Production of Fibrillar Material in Response to Stress

If one examines either bone or skin one finds that fibrillar material, such as collagen, is distributed along the lines of tension. Bone subjected to tensile forces is strengthened by such deposition. The skin similarly responds to external forces by the formation of callus and during development by the deposition of elastin fibres along the lines of Langer. Space medicine has drawn attention to the manner in which weightlessness leads to degradation of collagen in both skin and bone. The phenomenon has also been noted in paraplegia. Osteoporosis is a consequence of both weightlessness and paralysis (Claus-Walker *et al.*, 1982). Wounds of the skin or bone heal more firmly and thus resist forces tending to separate the wound edge if they are not too firmly splinted (Arem and Madden, 1976; Urschel *et al.*, 1988). Sutures or inflexible templates supporting a wound edge have been used to reduce the density of scars.

CELLULAR RESPONSES TO MECHANICAL FORCES

Microscopically, when cells are subjected to stress, tending to distort, they lay down more cytoskeleton in the form of actin filaments (White *et al.*, 1983; Drenckhahn *et al.*, 1984) (Figure 11.1). Further modifications are the laying down of keratin or the production of actin myosin. No skeleton is effective unless it is stabilised by attachment to its surrounds and there are numerous materials now recognised that act as adhesive materials on cell membranes. Vinculin and integrin glue the cytoskeleton, whereas materials like fibronectin and laminin are extracellular glues (Singer, 1982) Ingber and Jamieson (1985) described how strength and pliability in moving cells is determined by struts of cytoskeleton attached quite firmly

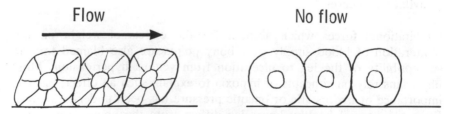

Figure 11.1   The endothelial cell develops a cytoskeleton in response to the forces of blood flow, which tends to distort and tear the cell from its anchorage

to the cell membrane, the attachment being the principal source of strength. However, moving cells need to be able to disattach themselves equally effectively. Ryan (1985, 1988) has emphasised the need for proteases to dissolve cell glues and thus allow the cell to disattach itself. In the literature on cell biology there are numerous observations on the responses of cells to stress and there is a clear relationship between cell attachment, cell shape, migration and mitosis. Curtis and Seehar (1978) have emphasised that oscillatory tensions applied to cells stimulates mitotic rates. Delvoye *et al.* (1987) described how tensile forces applied to fibroblasts influence collagen production, depending on whether the forces are isotonic or isometric. Chondrocytes produce more proteoglycans when they are subjected to mechanical stresses (De Witt *et al.*, 1984). Myotubules *in vitro* develop hypertrophy when subject to stretching (Vandenburgh and Kaufman, 1979) and there are several other observations of this nature (Maroudas, 1973; Folkman and Moscona, 1978; Ryan, 1985). In the field of embryogenesis it is well recognised that tensile forces converted into tractional forces have an influence on extracellular matrix and the polarisation of cells (Beloussov *et al.*, 1975; Harris *et al.*, 1981; Stopack and Harris, 1982). Binderman *et al.* (1984), studying bones, showed that both tensile forces and electric stimulation of different populations of bone cells, specifically triggered the adenyl cyclase system. They postulated a mechano-receptor on the cell membrane of osteoblasts.

Control of Fibrin Deposition

Deposition of fibrin is a fine balance between systems, tending to encourage coagulation and systems, such as fibrinolysis, which remove fibrin. There is a theory that on the internal surface of the vessel wall, slipperiness depends on the fibrin wall film which is constantly deposited and constantly removed (Copley, 1959). It is fibrinolysis which protects the vessels from coagulation. Injury to the epidermis, especially by shearing forces, is associated with a reduction of fibrinolytic activity in the upper dermis (Nishioka and Ryan, 1971) (Figure 11.2). There are several studies which suggest that fibrin can act as a scaffold in wound healing and that extracellular glues such as fibronectin are important for cell migration. Remoulding of a fibrin scaffold is important also for wound healing. Fibrin has to be removed before complete healing can occur. It has been argued that anchorage dependence of cells is inversely proportional to plasminogen activator production (Pollack *et al.*, 1974). One has only to add a minute amount of a protease such as trypsin to cause cells *in vitro* to disaggregate and to impede cell migration. There is also a concept that cells tend to move in the direction of a more sticky surface and away from areas that are slippery (Oster *et al.*, 1983). On the other hand, a dense fibrin clot

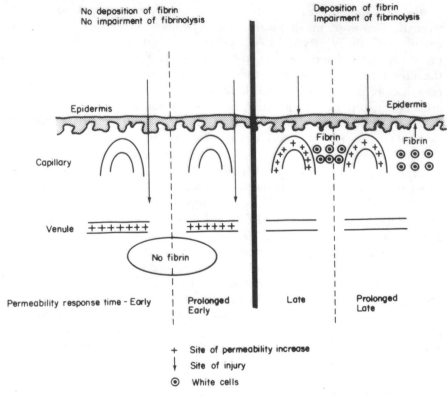

+ Site of permeability increase
↓ Site of injury
⊙ White cells

Figure 11.2 Injury to the epidermis (arrows), particularly from shearing strain, causes deposition of fibrin and impairment of fibrinolysis in the upper dermis. Injury of a similar degree but located deep in the dermis produces no deposition of fibrin and no impairment of fibrinolysis

can act as a barrier to the invasion of granulation tissue.

Currently, great interest in the new hydrocolloid dressings as promoters of healing has led to an investigation of their potential fibrinolytic activity, removing dense fibrin clots and allowing granulation tissue to develop more profusely (Lydon *et al.*, 1988). It was because the control of fibrinolysis seemed to be such an integral part of wound healing that Ryan and his colleagues decided to examine the role of mechanical forces in the control of proteolysis. Initially, Ryan and Barnhill (1983) studied whether wound contraction was in itself a stimulus to angiogenesis. In the belief that inhibitors of fibrinolysis might be produced by cells subjected to forces of stretch, Masuzawa and Ryan (1985) studied the effects of cell distortion on the production of urokinase inhibitor. Using centrifugation to distort fibroblasts, they observed that only 6 hours of mild centrifugation changed the behaviour of the fibroblast in tissue culture for many days thereafter. Such cells grew less fast and produced large amounts of inhibitors of urokinase. Masuzawa, Cherry and Ryan (1985) then studied the effect of skin expansion *in vivo* and found that this too caused fibroblasts to produce large amounts of intracellular inhibitor of urokinase. It thus seems possible that forces tending to distort the skin, such as shearing forces or pressure, might well stimulate the production of inhibitors of proteases (Ryan, 1988). This could contribute to the kind of coagulation necrosis that is seen in the early stages of a pressure sore.

TISSUE ORGANISATION AND THE TRANSMISSION OF MECHANICAL FORCES

The epidermis is attached to the dermis by a complex basement lamina which includes anchoring fibrils and extracellular glue-like materials. Shearing forces are transmitted along fibres orientated along lines of tension. How cells such as the epidermal or fibroblasts feel such forces depends on their relationship to such fibres and whether at points of attachment distorting forces transduce chemical signals. For a cell membrane to feel distortion, there must be attachment. Other factors which will influence the transmission of mechanical forces will be the flexibility of fibres, the contractility of cells and the swelling of the ground substance in an inflexible fibrillar environment (Ryan, 1988) (Figure 11.3). It is for this

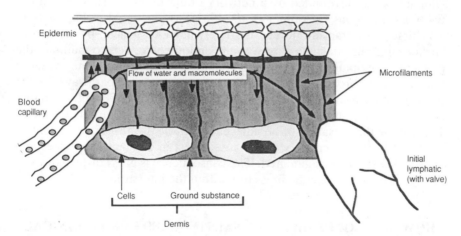

Figure 11.3 Distorting forces on the cell membrane, influenced by attachment of microfilaments, are affected by the flexibility of microfilaments and the swelling of the ground substance, as well as by contractility of cells. Flow of water and macromolecules from the blood vessels along the elastin pathway into the lymphatic also is to be taken into account. Such oedema-provoking phenomena raise the hydrostatic pressure and thus stress the solid elements of the tissues. It is postulated that such stressing is the mechanism whereby vital forces are distributed to all epithelial tissues

reason that it matters whether a tissue is composed of long or short, flexible or inflexible, fibres of collagen, and it is in this way that collagen types, of which there are now many, may influence the responses of the tissues. In tissues subjected repeatedly to mechanical forces, the fibroblasts become more contractile, and indeed become known as myofibroblasts. The contractility of cells attached to inflexible fibres may lead to the transmission of forces further afield. In such an environment, the capacity of hyaluronic acid to swell can be an important factor in determining how much tension is felt in the tissue. Since other glycosaminoglycans may influence swelling pressure, the presence of materials like chondroitin sulphate, heparan sulphate or dermatan sulphate becomes important.

Two other components that are important are the blood vessel and the lymphatic, because ultimately it is a balance between delivery of water and macromolecules to the tissue and their removal which determines the oncotic and hydrostatic pressure of the tissues (Ryan, 1988). If a tissue becomes over-hydrated and tension builds up, then for the reasons stated above, this could contribute to proteolysis inhibition.

In the study of decubitus ulcers, very little attention has been given to lymphatics and yet almost no other system is as sensitive to pressure and shearing strain (see Chapter 16). The lymphatics are essential for the removal of macromolecules and if they do not function then lymphoedema supervenes and the tissues may suffocate from their own effluent. The lymphatics are surrounded by a network of elastin in the skin, which has two main functions (Mortimer *et al.*, 1983), as illustrated in Figure 11.4. The first is to transmit forces to the lymphatic, which, by numerous anchoring fibrils attaching elastin to the endothelium, acts to maintain the patency of the pathways into the lymphatic. There is also some evidence that the large, broad fibres of elastin are low-resistance pathways for the passage of macromolecules through the tissues (Hauck, 1982). Lymphatics function almost entirely by responding to movement in their environment. This can be the pulsation of an adjacent arteriole or muscle movement or massage. Responsiveness of lymphatics is lost in oedematous tissues and elastin may become fragmented. The consequence is gross disturbances of the hydrostatic and oncotic pressures within the interstitium.

HOW ARE BIOCHEMICAL SIGNALS INDUCED BY MECHANICAL FORCES?

The suggestion that biochemical signals are transduced by mechanical forces, which derive mainly from studies of bone, needs to be studied alongside observations on the behaviour of the cell membrane subjected to distortion (Figure 11.5). There is, in fact, considerable fluidity within the cell membrane and certain components can be displaced by mechanical

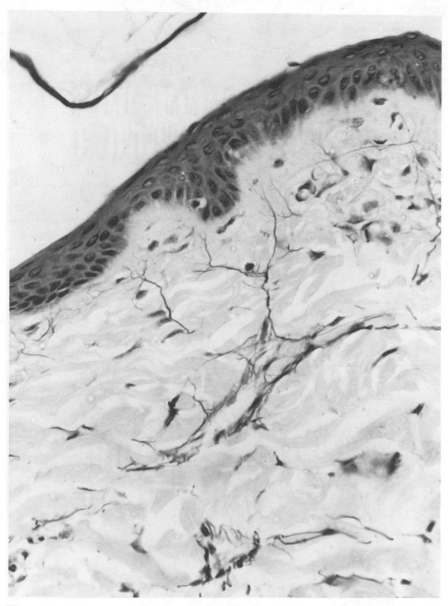

Figure 11.4 The lymphatic vessel is the principal exit pathway from the tissues of macromolecules, cells, and excess fluid. The elastin network that surrounds the lymphatic in the skin is essentially an external skeleton necessary for lymphatic function

distortion. There is some evidence that displacement of cholesterol leads to changes in the rigidity of the cell membrane, and that in addition certain proteins that are attached to the cell membrane may be switched to the cell

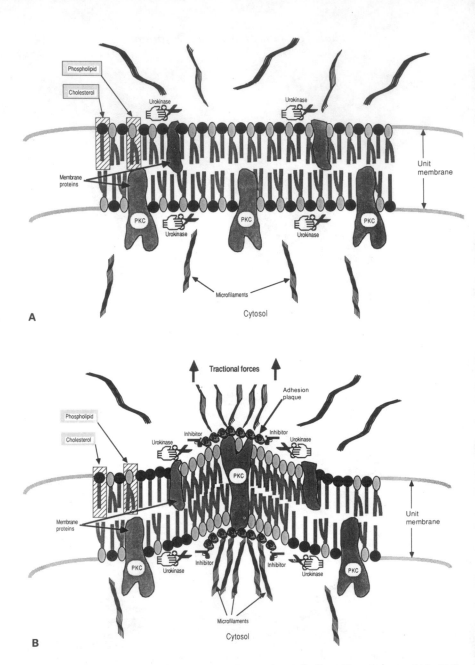

Figure 11.5 Hypothetic concept of the action of distorting forces. (A) Cell membrane not subjected to distorting forces, proteinkinase C (PKC) lies in the cytosol, and there is no phosphorlylation of adhesive material and no inhibition of urokinase and thus no attachment to microfilaments. (B) It is conceivable that tractional forces that alter the composition of cell membrane by displacing cholesterol switch proteinkinase C into action. Cell glues such as vinculin are phosphorylated, and adhesion plaques are formed only if at the same time there is inhibition of urokinase. Attachment of microfilaments is a consequence

Inhibitor Activity

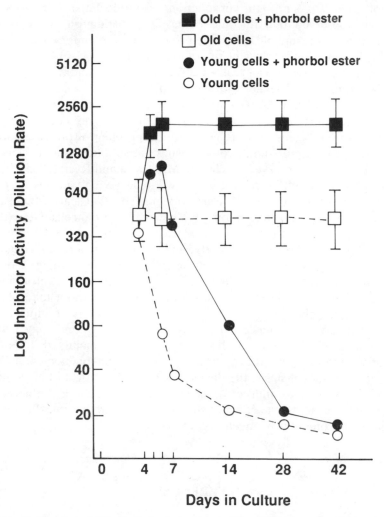

Figure 11.6 The addition of phorbal ester to fibroblasts in cell culture causes a significant increase in the production of intracellular inhibitor of urokinase. This is sustained in old cells but transient in young cells

surface when the cell membrane is distorted and the fluid elements are displaced (reviewed by Ryan, 1988). One enzyme in which this may occur is proteinkinase C. There are a number of reasons why this enzyme may be of particular interest. For one thing, it is required for the phosphorylation of the intercellular glue, vinculin, which binds actin fibres to the cell membrane (Pollanen *et al.*, 1988; Hebert and Baker, 1988). Another is that phorbol esters, which are much used in the study of cell behaviour, have proteinkinase C as their substrate. Horiuchi and Ryan (1987), using phorbol esters to study the production of intracellular inhibitors of urokinase, observed that it could be used to distinguish between the behaviour of young and old cells. The production of inhibitors is sustained in old cells but is only transient in young cells (Figure 11.6). Embryonic and newborn cells require a greater degree of flexibility and it is important that they should not be able to sustain production of inhibitors when stimulated by mechanical forces, whereas old cells and old tissues require a certain degree of stability so that remoulding processes are not too active. This concept too seems to be relevant to the problem of pressure sores, which are hardly a problem in young tissues but so much of a problem in the elderly. Several observers, including Masuzawa and Ryan (1985), have noted that old fibroblasts grow more slowly than young and this may be related to the inhibitor story (Masuzawa *et al.*, 1988). Clearly, there are also many other factors determining the behaviour of old cells. Nevertheless, it is conceivable that mechanical stresses produce a more sustained inhibition of proteolysis in the elderly, and this may encourage a coagulation response in ischaemic skin and at the same time delay healing. Wound repair always requires a certain degree of flexibility in the proteolytic system, and if this is lost then remoulding processes cannot take place. Ryan (1976) emphasised in a monograph on microvascular injury that tissues that have experienced previous injury of any kind may suffer exhaustion of fibrinolysis. In this text, which was mainly devoted to vasculitis, attention was drawn to the Shwartzmann phenomenon, the effect of gravitational stasis, the delayed skin flap, the effect of cold and a variety of other kinds of injuries which can make the skin more vulnerable. To this might be added the effect of shearing strain and the transduction of inhibitors of proteolysis by mechanical forces.

REFERENCES

Arem, A. J. and Madden, J. W. (1976). Effects of stress on healing wounds: 1. Intermittent noncyclical tension. *J. Surg. Res.*, **20**, 93–102

Beloussov, L., Dorfman, J. and Cherdantzev, V. (1975). Mechanical stresses and morphological patterns in amphibian embryos. *J. Embryol. Exp. Morphol.*, **34**, 559–574

Binderman, I., Shimshoni, Z. and Somjen, D. (1984). Biochemical pathways involved in the translation of physical stimulus into biological message. *Calcif. Tissue Int.*, **36**, 582–585

Claus-Walker, J., Di Ferrante, N., Halstead, L. S. and Tavella, D. (1982). Connective tissue turnover in quadraplega. *Am. J. Phys. Med.*, **61**, 130–140

Copley, A. L., Steichele, D., Spradau, M. and Thorley, R. S. (1959). Anticoagulant action of fibrin surfaces on mammalian blood. *Nature*, **183**, 1683–1684

Curtis, A. S. G. and Seehar, G. M. (1978). The control of cell division by tension or diffusion. *Nature*, **274**, 52–53

De Witt, M. T., Handley, C. J., Oakes, B. W. and Lowther, D. A. (1984). *In vitro* response of chondrocytes to mechanical loading. The effect of short mechanical stress. *Connect. Tissue Res.*, **1297**, 97–109

Delvoye, P., Nusgens, B. and Lapiere, C. M. (1987). Regulation of metabolism of skin fibroblasts by mechanical tension. (Abstract.) *J. Invest Dermatol.*, **89**, 332

Drenckhahn, D., Wagner, J., Gess, T. and Franke, R. P. (1984). Actin filament stress fibres in human vascular endothelium *in situ* and *in vitro*; molecular composition; requirements for contraction, and response to experimental fluid shear stress. (Abstract.) *Int. J. Microcirc. Clin. Exp.*, **3**, 274

Folkman, J. and Moscona, A. (1978). Role of cell shape in growth control. *Nature*, **273**, 345–349

Harris, A. K., Stopak, D. and Wild, P. (1981). Fibroblast traction as a mechanism for collagen morphogenesis. *Nature*, **290**, 249–251

Hauck, G. (1982). The connective tissue space in view of lymphology. *Experientia*, **38**, 1121–1122

Hebert, C. A. and Baker, J. B. (1988). Linkage of extracellular plasminogen activator to the fibroblast cytoskeleton: collocation of cell surface urokinase with vinculin. *J. Cell Biol.*, **106**, 1241–1247

Horiuchi, Y. and Ryan, T. J. (1987). Phorbol ester stimulates urokinase-inhibitor synthesis by cultured human fibroblasts. *Br. J. Dermatol.*, **116**, 419–420

Ingber, D. E. and Jamieson, J. D. (1985). Cells as tensegrity structures: architectural regulation of histodifferentiation by physical forces transduced over basement membrane. In Anderson, L. C., Gaggmberg, C. G. and Ekblom, P. (eds), *Gene Expression During Normal and Malignant Differentiation*, Academic Press, New York, pp. 13–32

Lydon, M. J., Johnson, E. R., Scudder, C., Adams, S. A., Cherry, G., Heaf, D. J., Fairbrother, J. E. and Cederholm-Williams, S. A. (1988). Fibrinolytic activity of hydrocolloid dressing. In Ryan, T. J. (ed.), *Beyond Occlusion. Wound Care Proceedings*, Royal Society of Medicine Services Ltd, London, pp. 9–17

Maroudas, N. G. (1973). Growth of fibroblasts on linear and planar anchorages of limiting dimensions. *Exp. Cell Research*, **81**, 111

Masuzawa, M. and Ryan, T. J. (1985). Proteolysis and cell behaviour under the influence of physical force. *Int. J. Microcirc. Clin. Exp.*, **4**, 297

Masuzawa, M., Cherry, G. W. and Ryan, T. J. (1985). Cellular proteolytic metabolism of fibroblasts and stretched skin. *Int. J. Microcirc. Clin. Exp.*, **4**, 297

Masuzawa, M., Hamasaki, H., Nishioka, K., Nishiyama, S. and Ryan, T. J. (1988). Urokinase-inhibitor of human fibroblasts – correlation with cell growth. In Gaffney, P. J., Castellino, F. J., Plow, E. F. and Takada, A. (eds), *Fibrinolysis Current Prospects*, Libbey, London, pp. 119–124

Mortimer, P. S., Cherry, G. W., Jones, R. L., Barnhill, R. L. and Ryan, T. J. (1983). The importance of elastic fibres in skin lymphatics. *Br. J. Dermatol.*, **108**, 561–566

Mridha, M. and Odman, S. (1985). Characterization of subcutaneous edema by mechanical impedance measurements. *J. Invest. Dermatol.*, **85**, 575–578

Nishioka, K. and Ryan, T. J. (1971). Inhibitors and proactivators of fibrinolysis in human epidermis. *Br. J. Dermatol.*, **85**, 561–565

Oster, G. F., Murray, J. D. and Harris, A. K. (1983). Mechanical aspects of mesenchymal morphogenesis. *J. Embryol. Exp. Morphol.*, **78**, 83–125

Pollack, R., Risser, R. and Conlon, S. (1974). Plasminogen activator production accompanies loss of anchorage regulation in transformation of primary rat embryo cells by Simian virus 40. *Proc. Natl Acad. Sci. USA*, **71**, 4792–4796

Pollanen, J., Hedman, K., Nielsen, L. S., Dano, K. and Vaheri, A. (1988). Ultrastructural localization of plasma membrane-associated urokinase-type plasminogen activator at focal contacts. *J. Cell Biol.*, **106**, 87–95

Ryan, T. J. (ed.) (1976). *Microvascular Injury* (Vol. 7, 'Major Problems in Dermatology'), Lloyd Luke Medical, London

Ryan, T. J. (1985). The Dowling Oration: Morphosis, occult forces and ectoplasm – the role of glues and proteolysis in skin disease. *Clin. Exp. Dermat.*, **10**, 507–522

Ryan, T. J. (1988). Biochemical consequences of mechanical forces generated by distention and distortion. *Am. J. Acad. Dermatol* (in press)

Ryan, T. J. and Barnhill, R. L. (1983). Physical factors and angiogenesis. In Nugent J. and O'Connor, M. (eds), *Development of the Vascular System*, Ciba Foundation Symposium, Pitman, London, pp. 80–94

Singer, I. I. (1982). Association of fibronectin and vinculin with focal contacts and stress fibers in stationary hamster fibroblasts. *J. Cell. Biol.*, **92**, 398–408

Stopak, D. and Harris, A. K. (1982). Connective tissue morphogenesis by fibroblast traction. I: Culture observations. *Dev. Biol.*, **90**, 383–398

Urschel, J. D., Scott, P. G. and Williams, T. G. (1988). The effect of mechanical stress on soft and hard tissue repair; a review. *Br. J. Plast. Surg.*, **41**, 182–186

Vandenburgh, H. and Kaufman, S. (1979). *In vitro* model for stretch-induced hypertrophy of skeletal muscle. *Science*, **203**, 265–268

White, G. E., Gimbrone, M. A. J. and Fujiwara, K. (1983). Factors influencing the expression of stress fibres in vascular endothelial cells *in situ*. *J. Cell. Biol.*, **2**, 416–424

12

Microvascular Mechanisms in Stasis and Ischaemia

C. C. Michel and Hilary Gillott

INTRODUCTION

When sufficient pressure is applied to the skin, the underlying blood vessels are occluded or partially occluded and oxygen and other nutrients are no longer delivered at a rate sufficient to satisfy the metabolic requirements of the tissues. To survive, the cells must draw upon their stores of energy. Without a circulation, the breakdown products of metabolism accumulate within the interstitial spaces and within the cells. As energy stores run out, the cellular processes begin to fail. Ionic gradients across cellular membranes begin to dissipate and the redistribution of fluid which may occur between the cells and extracellular spaces has consequences which in some situations render recovery impossible.

Usually vascular occlusion is short-lived and in regions of the skin such as the soles of the feet and the buttocks, short periods of occlusion are a necessary part of normal life. A short period of vascular occlusion is followed by a period of increased blood flow through the tissues which had been ischaemic. This increased blood flow after occlusion is called reactive hyperaemia. It is a consequence of a local regulatory mechanism whereby the arterioles are dilated and the resistance to blood flow is reduced. The same mechanism may operate to maintain blood flow through a tissue when an artery is partially occluded and the pressure difference which drives blood through the microcirculation is greatly reduced.

A rather different local regulatory mechanism operates when the veins are partially occluded. The rise in local venous pressure is accompanied by constriction of the arterioles, which reduces total blood flow and also minimises the rise in local microvascular pressure. This mechanism, the veni-arteriolar response, appears to be of considerable physiological importance in the limbs, where venous pressure may rise as venous return is hindered by gravity.

In this chapter we review these two local vascular responses. We also consider briefly the responses of the skin microcirculation to local compression and speculate on the changes which may occur when periods of occlusion are not relieved within a short period of time, owing to paralysis or immobility. Such changes are preliminary to the development of pressure sores.

REACTIVE HYPERAEMIA

Reactive hyperaemia is a phenomenon that can be demonstrated in the circulation of most tissues and organs. It has been investigated most extensively in the limbs of human subjects and experimental animals, but usually no distinction has been made between the contributing effects of muscle and skin circulations. Figure 12.1(a) shows the changes in blood flow through the human forearm which occur after a 3-minute period of occlusion. Blood flow has a maximal value immediately after the occlusion is released. Flow then declines exponentially to the control (pre-occlusion) value. If the arterial supply to the limb is cut off for more than 5 minutes, peak blood flow is maintained for a period as a high plateau before it declines exponentially to the pre-occlusion level (Figure 12.1(b)).

For occlusions of up to 5 minutes, the peak flow of hyperaemia correlates with the duration of vascular occlusion which preceded it. Attempts have also been made to correlate the increased blood flow during the reactive hyperaemia with the flow that would have occurred during the period of occlusion (the so-called 'blood flow debt'). Such correlations are approximate and may be abolished by certain experimental procedures. For example, Blair *et al.* (1959) were able to abolish reactive hyperaemia in the human forearm by partial occlusion of the brachial artery when total occlusion was released. The interpretation of experiments of this kind and the quantitative analysis of the changes in hyperaemic blood flow are of

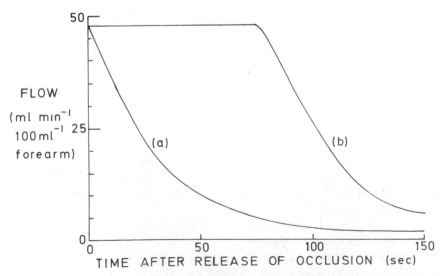

Figure 12.1 Changes in forearm blood flow after (a) 3 minutes' ischaemia, (b) 10 minutes' ischaemia. The cuff occluding arterial flow into the limb was released at zero time

considerable importance in understanding the underlying mechanisms.

We have described the fall in blood flow in reactive hyperaemia as exponential and indeed Dornhorst and Whelan (1953) found that their data on the human forearm was described by a single exponential decay. Recently Imms *et al.* (1988) have re-examined the question and found that in most of their subjects the decline in forearm blood flow with time following a period of occlusion could be described best by a composite of two exponentials. Imms *et al.* (1988) suggested that the two components of reactive hyperaemia might reflect different time constants for the reactions of the blood vessels of the skin and the muscle. This hypothesis can be tested by modern techniques and it is worth noting that in spite of intense interest up to 20 to 30 years ago, there is still much to be learnt about the quantitative phenomenology of reactive hyperaemia.

Reactive hyperaemia is most easily demonstrated in human limbs if the skin is warm. Post-occlusion hyperaemia is much reduced in a cooled limb. In a systematic investigation of the phenomenon in the hand immersed in water at varying temperatures, Catchpole and Jepson (1955) found that average peak flow post-occlusion rose from 3.05 to 9.8 ml 100 ml^{-1} min^{-1} of tissue between 15 °C and 25 °C, increasing to 19.8 ml 100 ml^{-1} min^{-1} at 30 °C.

Reactive hyperaemia was shown to be independent of connections with the central nervous system at the end of the last century. Bier (1897) reported that while amputating limbs he divided the nerves and flesh first, leaving the main artery and vein intact. Under these conditions temporary occlusion of the artery was followed by the usual hyperaemia (Greenfield, 1963). Subsequently, Lewis and Grant (1925) demonstrated that skin which had been rendered anaesthetic by lesion of the main nerves reacted similarly to adjacent skin which retained normal innervation after a period of vascular occlusion. Eichna and Wilkins (1941) reported that in patients with chronically denervated and wasted forearms, the peak blood flow during reactive hyperaemia was 26 per cent greater than that in the normal innervated limb when the flows were expressed in terms of ml per 100 ml of tissue. The peak flow and duration of the reactive hyperaemia has also been found to be similar in normal and chronically sympathectomised limbs (Freeman, 1935). Since neither acute nor chronic denervation appear to affect the maximal blood flows that are achieved in reactive hyperaemia, it is safe to conclude that its mechanism is independent of vasomotor nerves.

Although there is some evidence that a lowered transmural pressure difference across the walls of the arterioles might contribute to the vasodilatation of reactive hyperaemia, it is generally believed that the vasodilatation results either from the action of agents released from the anoxic tissues, or from the lack of O_2 itself, or from a combination of O_2 lack and locally released vasodilator agents. This general view is supported in the broadest sense by the demonstration that venous blood collected during reactive hyperaemia has vasodilator properties. That oxygen lack alone may contribute in a major way to the hyperaemic vasodilatation is supported by the vasodilator effects of anoxic blood and by an experiment of Fairchild *et al.* (1966). These workers perfused the hind limb of a dog either with the animal's own arterial (oxygenated) blood or with blood which had been equilibrated with N_2 and 5 per cent CO_2 in a blood–gas equilibrator. A period of occlusion of arterial inflow to the limb was followed by a hyperaemic response, which decayed exponentially if arterial blood entering the limb was oxygenated. If, during the period of occlusion, however, the arterial inflow was changed from oxygenated blood to anoxic blood, the same peak blood flow was attained when flow was restored and it remained high and showed no attenuation with time. From this Fairchild *et al.* (1966) concluded that the principal factor responsible for the vasodilation was the local PO_2 in the tissues. They argued that if the vasodilation resulted from the action of a metabolite which was released from the ischaemic tissues and could be cleared in the blood, then the restoration of blood flow should have lowered its level in the tissues and blood flow should have subsequently been reduced. Fairchild *et al.* (1966) recognised that their results were open to alternative interpretations. The level of the vasodilatory agent in the vicinity of the arterioles might be determined by the balance between its rate of release from the anoxic cells (a process determined by anoxia) and its rate of clearance by the blood and reuptake into the cells in the presence of oxygen. Thus restoration of flow with anoxic blood might have resulted in only a modest fall in the tissue levels of the metabolite. Whereas a modest fall in the tissue level of the hypothetical vasodilator agent might be expected to reduce blood flow when the peak flow is sub-maximal, when vasodilatation is maximal, reduction in the level of the vasodilator agent might have little effect. Such a mechanism could well be responsible for the plateau of peak flow which is seen after prolonged periods of ischaemia in the human forearm.

The plateau of peak flow after prolonged ischaemia may be regarded as evidence against the local PO_2 being the sole factor responsible for the hyperaemia. The observation that the PO_2 of the venous blood may rise above its pre-occlusion value during the period of hyperaemia is additional evidence for this view. The identity of the vasodilator agent remains unclear, though there have been and still remain many possible candidates for the role. Lewis (1927) believed that histamine was responsible but quite apart from less direct evidence, the hypothesis moved into the background when Emmelin and Emmelin (1947) showed that reactive hyperaemia can be demonstrated in the presence of high levels of antihistamines. More recently, prostaglandin-like substances have been suggested as the vaso-dilatory mediator in reactive hyperaemia and there is evidence that the hyperaemic response is attenuated after pre-treatment with indomethacin (a prostaglandin synthesis inhibitor). In the coronary circulation, Berne (1980) has argued strongly for adenosine as the vasodilator of reactive hyperaemia and recent evidence for its accumulation in endothelial cells has added further interest in the adenosine hypothesis. Adenosine triphosphate (ATP) has vasodilator properties which recently have been closely linked to the release of EDRF (endothelial derived relaxing factor) from endothelial cells, and both prostacyclin and EDRF itself are possible candidates. As the pharmacology of these agents develops it seems most likely that an understanding of their physiological roles will soon emerge. At present it seems that there is a sufficient number of candidates to act as vasodilator substances in reactive hyperaemia. It could be that the total response is the result of the action of several agents and the type of agent which predominates varies in different vascular beds.

THE VENI-ARTERIOLAR RESPONSE

The hypothesis that an increase in the transmural pressure difference across the walls of the resistance vessels might lead to their further constriction, and that a reduction in transmural pressure might lead to vasodilation, was suggested by Bayliss (1902). Although it periodically received attention during the subsequent half-century, it was only in the late 1940s that convincing experimental evidence for a mechanism of this kind became apparent. Folkow (1949) demonstrated that in different vascular beds changes in resistance accompanied changes in the pressure gradients across the bed. Working on the responses of the intestinal circulation, Johnson (1964) showed that increases in intravascular pressure invoked increases in arteriolar resistance but that the response was much more sensitive to increases in venous pressure (which would raise the pressure at the capillary end of the arterioles) than to increases in arterial pressure. The phenomenon was beautifully illustrated in the microcirculation by Johnson and Wayland (1967), who demonstrated the effects of raising and lowering arterial and venous pressure on red-cell velocity in single microvessels.

Evidence for a phenomenon of this kind in human subjects was reported in a series of studies by Henriksen and his colleagues (1977). Measuring local blood flow by the ^{133}Xe clearance technique, he demonstrated how increases in venous pressure in the limbs, resulting from either posture or from venous occlusion, led to an increase in the local vascular resistance. Raising the limb above heart level to reduce the intravascular pressures gave rise to a fall in local vascular resistance. Direct evidence that the increase in resistance with increased venous pressure was pre-capillary was provided by Levick and Michel (1978), who measured capillary pressures in the hands and feet by micropuncture, together with the local venous pressure, as venous pressure was raised either by lowering the extremity below the heart or by partial occlusion of the veins.

Henriksen's studies (1977) on a patient with a long-standing unilateral sympathectomy and on another patient before and immediately after a sympathectomy, led him to draw attention to the importance of sympathetic nerves in the response. The patient whom he investigated before and immediately after the sympathectomy retained the response of an increase in vascular resistance to an increase in local venous congestion immediately after his operation, but the response was lost 3–4 days post-operatively. The patient with a long-standing unilateral sympathectomy showed no response in his sympathectomised limb but a normal response in the contralateral arm. Henriksen (1977) suggested that the response was dependent upon the sympathetic nerves but not their central connections. An axon reflex of sympathetic fibres conveyed information of venous distension directly to the arterioles causing them to contract. In support of his hypothesis, Henriksen (1977) reported a series of ingenious experiments on the clearance of ^{133}Xe from subcutaneous tissue on the forearm.

The veni-arterial response serves to minimise the rise in microvascular pressure as venous pressure rises, particularly in lower limbs during quiet standing (Mellander *et al.*, 1964; Levick and Michel, 1978; Sjersen *et al.*, 1981). The protection of the tissues under these normal physiological conditions ultimately depends upon the importance of voluntary movements, which keep down the venous pressure with remarkable efficiency when the venous valves are competent.

PARTIAL ARTERIAL OCCLUSION AND VENOUS CONGESTION

Partial occlusion (or complete occlusion) of the arterial supply to an area of tissue may occur temporarily as a result of compression or more permanently as a result of large vessel disease. If the occlusion is partial then the distal areas of the vascular bed show a compensatory reduction in vascular resistance. The phenomenon has been demonstrated in experimental animals where a reduction of the perfusion pressure in a localised region of the circulation is accompanied by a reduction in the vascular resistance of that region. In this way it is possible to maintain the nutritive flow to a tissue in the face of falling perfusion pressure, the phenomenon of autoregulation of blood. It is likely that the mechanisms responsible for the decreased vascular resistance are those involved in reactive hyperaemia.

When partial occlusion of the arteries is a consequence of large vessel disease, longer-term changes in the microvasculature may occur with increased vascularisation. This, in part, may account for the prolonged hyperaemic response which is reported to occur in the affected tissues after the occlusion has been surgically removed. The hyperaemia in this circumstance may persist for weeks.

Venous congestion may occur in immobilised limbs below heart level or as a result of venous occlusion or valvular incompetence. While the rise of microvascular pressure that accompanies any condition where venous pressure is raised is attenuated by the veni-arteriolar response, microvascular pressure is inevitably increased. Fluid is continually filtered from the microvasculature into the tissue and under conditions of low plasma flow the haematocrit and plasma protein concentration in venous blood are greatly increased. Thus in healthy subjects sitting voluntarily with their feet held still a metre below heart level, the haematocrit of the venous blood leaving the feet rises from an average of 42 per cent to 56 per cent over 40 min and total plasma protein concentration rises from $6.8 \, g \, dl^{-1}$ to $9.6 \, g \, dl^{-1}$ (68 to 96 mg ml^{-1}) (Moyses *et al.*, 1987). Plasminogen activator is released under these conditions and of considerable interest is failure of the leukocytes and platelets to appear in the venous blood in numbers which would be appropriate to the reduced blood volume. It is inferred that leukocytes, particularly the monocytes and neutrophils, accumulate in the microcirculation during venous congestion. Their activation here with release of proteolytic enzymes and generation of free radicals could be responsible for tissue damage following venous congestion.

MICROVASCULAR RESPONSES TO TISSUE COMPRESSION

If the skin is compressed over a localised area, then, depending upon the magnitude of the applied pressure, the underlying vasculature may be occluded or partly occluded. Romanus (1976) observed the microcirculation in the hamster cheek pouch as the external pressure was raised first to between 30 and 45 mmHg (4–6 kPa) and then to 60 mmHg (8 kPa). The initial effect of compressing the tissue to between 30 mmHg and 45 mmHg was to arrest the microcirculation. Then, after a variable period of time, the circulation restarted in some parts of the preparation but microvascular flow was slow and 'jerky'. When a pressure of 60 mmHg (8 kPa) was applied to the preparation the circulation stopped and did not resume until the pressure was reduced. Occlusion of the circulation for 3–3½ hours resulted in disturbances of the microvasculature during recovery. One hour after the pressure was reduced, bleeding was observed from some microvessels and thrombus formation in others. Cooling the tissues to 22 °C during the period of occlusion protected the microcirculation from these disturbances during reperfusion.

This qualitative description of partial recovery of flow in tissues under moderate degrees of compression is borne out by indirect quantitative measurements. Thus Holloway *et al.* (1976) measured the early effects of tissue loading on the clearance of ^{133}Xe from the skin on the volar aspect of the forearm and in the parasacral region. Flow was diminished by an applied pressure of 10 mmHg (1.3 kPa) but there was little further reduction in flow until the applied pressure exceeded 30 mmHg (4 kPa). With further loading flow diminished, becoming very small when pressure reached 60 mmHg (8 kPa). It is possible that if the authors had made measurements after longer periods of tissue loading, they might have observed higher flows at pressures lower than 45 mmHg. Bader (1989) has reported that after the initial fall in tissue PO_2 that follows tissue loading, a limited rise in PO_2 may occur. It would seem that the mechanisms responsible for reactive hyperaemia are operating under these conditions in response to partial occlusion of the microvasculature; indeed they are probably also operating to maintain blood flow under conditions of light compression in the experiments of Holloway *et al.* (1976).

A rather different effect of compression upon microvascular flow has been described by Nielsen (1982). He examined the effects of compressing the tissues of the lower leg of a subject with a cuff at a pressure of 60 mmHg (8 kPa) upon the clearance of ^{133}Xe from the underlying subcutaneous tissue and muscle. Flow was reduced in both tissues, the reduction being less severe in muscle. Elevation of the local venous pressure, however, increased subcutaneous blood flow without altering clearance from muscle. It is concluded that a major factor in reducing the flow to the subcutaneous tissue is the compression of the veins and venules, and that the raised venous pressure raised their conductance to a greater extent than it reduced the driving pressure for perfusion.

REPERFUSION FAILURE AND REPERFUSION INJURY

When an arterial obstruction is relieved after a prolonged period of ischaemia, the microcirculation may fail to reperfuse, or perfusion may be at a level well below normal. Observations *in vivo* in experimental animals reveal areas of stasis with columns of closely packed red cells obstructing the capillaries and venules. In some cases, one or more leukocytes can be seen at the head of the plug and many observations suggest that the leukocytes may be responsible for obstructing the microvessels under these circumstances. We noted earlier that during venous congestion, leukocytes appear to accumulate within the microvasculature. Direct observations on microvasculature of muscle in experimental animals in a state of haemorrhagic shock have revealed the sluggish movement of leukocytes and their arrest within the smallest microvessels, blocking the flow (Bagge *et al.*, 1980). If the circulation is reduced or arrested by external pressure then damage is likely to occur to the endothelial cells, which constitute the walls of the capillaries. If flow is reduced, leukocytes will adhere to the damaged sites and where the endothelium has been breached, platelets adhere to the exposed basement membrane and trigger the cascade of coagulation reactions, leading to obstruction by microthrombi. Damaged endothelial cells become 'sticky' and opposing cells brought into contact by external pressure may be loosely bonded and precipitate microvascular occlusion. Endothelium releases a range of substances, some of which act as dilators and some as constrictors to the neighbouring smooth muscle. If the balance of constrictors and dilators is disturbed by endothelial damage then the vasoconstrictor effects may predominate and overide the normal dilatory mechanisms.

Two processes common to all cells deprived of their energy supply might be at work and prevent reperfusion. The gradients of ions across membranes both within cells and separating cells from their extracellular environment are maintained by active energy requiring 'pumps'. A reduction in energy supply slows or stops the pumps and the ion gradients begin to dissipate. Normally cells are in osmotic equilibrium with the extracellular fluids, but as the ion gradients run down, so more ions enter the cells than leave them. The cells swell as water is drawn into them to maintain osmotic equilibrium. If the tissue is contained within a relatively rigid capsule, the swollen cells may compress and occlude the microvessels, preventing reperfusion. Such a mechanism could well be responsible for the 'no-flow phenomenon' of renal perfusion and for the compartmental syndrome responsible for the necrosis of muscle which follows ischaemia of the forearm and lower leg. Of the intracellular ionic concentrations which change during ischaemia, most devastating in its consequences is the rise of intracellular Ca^{2+}. Ca^{2+} ions are regulators of a wide variety of intracellular events from the activation of contractile mechanisms to the activation of proteolytic enzymes and the onset of autolysis. It could be that after prolonged ischaemia the intracellular Ca^{2+} of the smooth muscle cells of the feeding arterioles rises sufficiently for them to contract irreversibly, a sort of vascular *rigor mortis* which renders reperfusion impossible.

It is also recognised that after prolonged ischaemia reperfusion itself may promote tissue damage. When oxygen is reintroduced into ischaemic tissues, the transformation of certain enzymes and substrates leads to the formation of superoxides, oxygen free radicals which have a damaging effect on a variety of biomolecular structures. Superoxides are released in bursts by activated phagocytic cells but their generation during reperfusion appears to be related to the appearance of significant levels of hypoxanthine and xanthine oxidase in the tissues. In the presence of oxygen and xanthine oxidase, the hypoxanthine is converted into xanthine with liberation of hydrogen peroxide and superoxide. The origin of the hypoxanthine is probably ATP, the ubiquitous utilisable store of energy in all cells. In the absence of an energy supply the ATP is broken down to adenosine, then to inosine and finally to hypoxanthine. The xanthine oxidase is derived from xanthine dehydrogenase, an interconversion which results from a rise in intracellular Ca^{2+} which activates the appropriate protease.

Thus a range of different processes which occur during prolonged ischaemia may serve to prevent adequate reperfusion or promote tissue damage when reperfusion occurs.

ACKNOWLEDGEMENT

We wish to thank the Chest, Heart and Stroke Association for a scholarship to HG.

REFERENCES

Bader, D. L. (1989). Effects of compressive loading regimens on tissue viability, this volume, pp. 191–201

Bagge, U., Amundson, B. and Lauritzen, C. (1980). White cell deformability and plugging of skeletal muscle capillaries in haemorrhagic shock. *Acta Physiologica Scandinavica*, **180**, 159–163

Bayliss, W. M. (1902). On the local reactions of the arterial wall to changes of internal pressure. *Journal of Physiology*, **28**, 220–231

Berne, R. M. (1980). The role of adenosine in the regulation of coronary blood flow. *Circulation Research*, **47**, 807–813

Bier, A. (1897). Die Enstehung des Collateralkreislauf. I, Die arterielle Collateral-kreislauf. *Archiv für pathologische Anatomie und Physiologie*, **147**, 257–293

Blair, D. A., Glover, W. E. and Roddie, I. A. C. (1959). The abolition of reactive and post-exercise hyperaemia in the forearm by temporary restriction of arterial inflow. *Journal of Physiology*, **148**, 648–658

Catchpole, B. N. and Jepson, R. P. (1955). Hand and finger blood flow. *Clinical Science*, **14**, 109–120

Dornhorst, A. C. and Whelan, R. F. (1953). The blood flow in the muscle following exercise and circulatory arrest: the influence of reduction in effective local blood pressure, of arterial hypoxia and adrenaline. *Clinical Science*, **12**, 33–40

Eichna, L. W. and Wilkins, R. W. (1941). Blood flow to the forearm and calf. II, Reactive hyperaemia: factors influencing the blood flow during the vasodilatation following ischaemia. *Bulletin of Johns Hopkins Hospital*, **68**, 450–476

Emmelin, K. and Emmelin, N. (1947). Histamine and reactive hyperaemia. *Acta Physiologica Scandanavica*, **14**, 16–18

Fairchild, H. M., Ross, J. and Guyton, A. C. (1966). Failure of recovery from reactive hyperaemia in the absence of oxygen. *American Journal of Physiology*, **210**, 490–492

Folkow, B. (1949). Intravascular pressure as a factor regulating the tone of the small vessels. *Acta Physiologica Scandinavica*, **17**, 289–310

Freeman, N. E. (1935). The effect of temperature on the rate of blood flow in the normal and in the sympathectomised hand. *American Journal of Physiology*, **113**, 384–398

Greenfield, A. D. M. (1963). The circulation through the skin. In Hamilton, W. F. (ed.), *Handbook of Physiology: Circulation*, Section 2, Vol. II, American

Physiological Society, Washington DC, pp. 1325–1351

Henriksen, O. (1977). Local sympathetic reflex mechanism in regulation of blood flow in human subcutaneous adipose tissue. *Acta Physiologica Scandinavica* (suppl.), **450**, 7–48

Holloway, G. A., Daly, C. H., Kennedy, D. and Chimoskey, J. (1976). Effects of external pressure loading on human skin blood flow measured by ^{133}Xe clearance. *Journal of Applied Physiology*, **40**, 597–600

Imms, F. J., Lee, Wew-Sen and Ludlow, P. G. (1988). Reactive hyperaemia in the human forearm. *Quarterly Journal of Experimental Physiology*, **73**, 203–215

Johnson, P. C. (1964). Origin, localisation, and homeostatic significance of autoregulation in the intestine. *Circulation Research*, **14**, **15**, Suppl. 1, 225–232

Johnson, P. C. and Wayland, H. (1967). Regulation of blood flow in single capillaries. *American Journal of Physiology*, **212**, 1405–1415

Levick, J. R. and Michel, C. C. (1978). The effects of position and skin temperature on the capillary pressures in the fingers and toes. *Journal of Physiology*, **274**, 97–109

Lewis, T. (1927). *The Blood Vessels of the Human Skin and their Responses*, Shaw, London

Lewis, T. and Grant, R. T. (1925). Observations upon reactive hyperaemia in man. *Heart*, **12**, 73–120

Mellander, S., Oberg, B. and Odelram, H. (1964). Vascular adjustments to increased transmural pressure in cat and man with special reference to shifts in capillary fluid transfer. *Acta Physiologica Scandinavica*, **61**, 34–48

Moyses, C., Cederholm-Williams, S. A. and Michel, C. C. (1987). Haemoconcentration and accumulation of white cells in the feet during venous stasis. *Internal Journal of Microcirculation: Clinical & Experimental*, **5**, 311–320

Nielsen, H. V. (1982). Effects of externally applied compression on blood flow in subcutaneous and muscle tissue in the human supine leg. *Clinical Physiology*, **2**, 447–457

Romanus, E. M. (1976). Microcirculatory reactions to controlled tissue ischaemia and temperature: A vital microscopic study on the hamster's cheek pouch. In Kenedi *et al. Bed Sore Biomechanics*, pp. 79–82

Sejrsen, P., Henriksen, O. and Paaske, W. P. (1981). Effect of orthostatic blood pressure changes upon capillary filtration–absorption rate in the human calf. *Acta Physiologica Scandinavica*, **111**, 287–291

13

The Metabolic Basis of Wound Healing

A. W. Goode

INTRODUCTION

From the earliest days man has had an understanding about the mechanisms of wound healing. Although early ideas may have been crude and imprecise, they contained a basic awareness of what may enhance or retard the healing process, without an awareness of the underlying mechanisms. Ambroise Paré (1510–90), the father of modern surgery, who found that watery dressings were kinder to wounds than hot oil, stated many times that 'Man treats but God cures.' Although we now understand much of the biochemical and metabolic processes involved in healing, the clinical management of wounds may still be criticised for a lack of scientific basis. This is in part because of incomplete knowledge of the healing process and cellular and metabolic constraints on complete healing, and in part because of the poor quality of clinical measurement of healing to study the validity of competing claims of efficacy.

After injury the body repairs damaged tissue (Peacock and van Winkle, 1976; Rudolph, 1980). Structure and function are restored by a series of complex cellular and biochemical events which ultimately result in the formation of scar tissue. The underlying mechanism will result in an aesthetically acceptable wound with the aid of the surgeon. When wound edges are apposed accurately, minimal granulation tissue forms, with a small thin scar resulting. By contrast, when there is skin loss or infection in the wound, then the edges are not apposed and healing must proceed by the formation of copious granulation tissue. This constitutes healing by secondary intention, which results in dense fibrous scar tissue. Accurate measurement of healing rates in secondary intention is now possible with the technique of stereophotogrammetry (Bulstrode et al., 1986).

BIOCHEMICAL COMPONENTS OF HEALING

The granulation tissue of healing wounds is concerned with the production of both collagen and ground substance. Collagen is the extracellular fibrous framework which gives form and strength to tissue. Collagen is synthesised in the fibroblast and eventually extruded into extracellular connective tissue spaces. The collagen monomer is rod-shaped with a molecular weight of 350 000. Collagen is synthesised from three polypeptide chains, the pro-alpha chains, each chain containing about one thousand amino acids, glycine occupying every third position along their length. Of the remaining amino acids approximately one-third are combinations of proline and hydroxyproline, each of which has inherent rigidity in its ring structure.

Within the basic structure there are several types of collagen which differ in amino acid sequence. Type I collagen consists of two identical alpha chains with a third chain (alpha 2) and is found in skin, tendon, bone and ligamentous tissues. Type II collagen occurs in cartilage and type III is found in foetal dermis, changing to type I after birth. Granulation tissue is mainly type I collagen but may initially be up to 30 per cent made up of type III, the proportion falling with maturation.

Immature protocollagen may accumulate in fibroblasts. The polypeptide chains are rich in the amino acids proline and lysine, which are hydroxylated by the enzymes prolyl- and lysyl-hydroxylase. This reaction depends upon oxygen, ferrous enzymes, and the reducing substances ascorbic acid and alpha-ketogluterate. Lack of these factors inhibits hydroxylation and in turn glycosylation, the next step in maturation, will not occur. In optimal conditions glycosylation will proceed stabilising the alpha chains into the right-handed triple-helix structure. This tropocollagen, which is held together by weak electrostatic forces, is soluble in weak salt solutions and so is extruded from the fibroblast. Tropocollagen disappears quickly with maturation, whereby cross-linkages occur between aldehyde-containing amino acids of one collagen molecule and other amino acids in another collagen molecule. Such cross-linkages transform soluble tropocollagen into a stronger, less soluble form, which undergoes constant turnover under the influence of tissue collagenases.

Ground substance is the amorphous matrix of connective tissue. It exists in a water-rich phase in equilibrium with a colloid-rich phase and contains water, electrolytes, glycoproteins and mucopolysaccharides. Complexes occur between proteins and polysaccharides, termed proteoglycans, that give special properties to the ground substance. A protein core of molecular weight 200 000 surrounded by radially placed linear polysaccharide chains of molecular weight 2000 produces chondroitin sulphate. There are other mucopolysaccharides (also known as glycosaminoglycans), chondroitin, dermatan sulphate, keratan sulphate and hyaluronic acid. Usually, ground substance is a thin gel and its viscoelastic properties are very important in the load-bearing function of articular cartilage. It is probable that the collagen molecule is stabilised by bonding with mucopolysaccharides.

THE PHASES OF HEALING

There are three phases of wound healing, as shown in Table 13.1.

Table 13.1 The phases of wound healing

Phase	Days	
I	1–4	The phase of inflammation
II	5–20	The phase of proliferation
III	20+	The phase of differentiation

The Phase of Inflammation (Phase I)

Initially, for up to 4 days the wound undergoes a sequence of events that is basically inflammatory (Dunphy and Udupa, 1955). Changes in local pressure and tension within the soft tissues result in a change in the distribution of charge on the collagen molecule. Capillaries dilate and fluid accumulates in the wound (Alexander and Meakins, 1971). This fluid contains fibrinogen so a fibrin clot forms and kinin and complement cascades are induced. Platelets exposed to collagen release ADP, 5-hydroxytryptamine, prostacyclins and thromboxane A. More platelets adhere, and, together with clotting factors, form a haemostatic plug. Epithelium grows rapidly across the wound surface (van Winkle, 1968). Thus, in phase I, the wound is held together by the inserted surgical sutures, if any, fibrin and a weak epithelial surface. During this phase the blood vessels initially undergo constriction which is then followed by vasodilatation under the influence of histamine from platelets and mast cells. The blood flow slows, white cells marginate to the vessel walls and permeability increases. The response and subsequent capillary engorgement are initiated and maintained by histamine, serotonin, the kinins and prostaglandins (Kellermyer and Graham, 1968). Red and white cells escape through the capillary walls and a coagulum of fibrin forms.

In 2–3 hours a network of fibrin surrounds a few lymphocytes and an increasing number of polymorphonuclear leucocytes. Neutrophils predominate for the first 2 days. Monocytes infiltrate at a slightly later time, being the predominant cell type by day 5. Neutrophils lyse and release cytoplasmic granules, while monocytes are phagocytic and ingest cellular debris. If antimacrophage serum is administered to a wound then there is a marked delay in wound healing, but impairment of neutrophil function has little discernible effect.

The Phase of Proliferation (Phase II)

By day 5, fibroblasts move into the wound in large numbers, probably from multipotential stem cells in local small capillaries (Grillo, 1964). The fibroblasts synthesise collagen and ground substance, which make a new fibrous connective tissue within the wound's fibrin meshwork (Hunt, 1974). In this phase, the wound requires large amounts of nutrients, particularly protein, vitamin C and trace elements, especially zinc, to allow conversion of proline to hydroxyproline. The wound becomes thickened and reddened because of the active dilated capillaries and collagen deposition. In the actively healing wound, collagen degradation occurs simultaneously with collagen synthesis (Cohen and Keiser, 1976). In malnutrition, the patients may be unable to synthesise adequate amounts of collagen to balance degradation, resulting in wound dehiscence. The earliest collagen fibrils are laid down as slender reticulum fibres. Thicker collagen then predominates, being laid down in the characteristic random manner of granulation tissue.

The Phase of Differentiation (Phase III)

There is no clear demarcation between phases II and III. Differentiation involves simultaneous collagen degradation and synthesis with a reduced rate of synthesis compared with phase II. The total collagen content of the wound remains unchanged. With differentiation there is a rationalisation of the copious blood vessels, many of which occlude and disappear. Randomly arranged collagen fibres are the principal feature of the scar, but with time considerable remodelling occurs. Even in this phase of wound healing inadequate nutrition or poor vascular perfusion may result in wound dehiscence.

   Wounds that have lost skin by excision, or trauma, or wounds that have opened, undergo two other mechanisms of natural wound healing, namely, contraction and epithelialisation.

Contraction

This is the mechanism by which wound edges are drawn together. The wound fills with granulation tissue, so called because in reflected light it has a cobblestone appearance, with a healthy pink hue. The multiple nodules are composed of new fibroblasts, capillaries and collagen. Within 3–4 days after injury, the wound edges begin to be drawn together (van Winkle, 1967) in those tissues which are pliable. Thus, in a chronic wound with surrounding fibrosis contraction is impeded, while anatomical sites, such as the ankle, pretibial aspect of the leg, and the forehead, also are unyielding, resisting natural contraction. Thus, chronic wounds are particularly common in these sites, and indeed if a surgeon in any site is unable to appose wound edges without undue force it is improbable that wound contraction will close the wound.

Collagen is not a contractile protein and the mechanism is cellular. The contractile cells in the granulation tissue are myofibrils, having the electron microscope characteristics of fibroblasts and smooth muscle cells (Gabbiani, 1971), and exhibit a pharmacological response to stimulation and relaxation. Myofibroblasts are found in burns, scars, Dupuytren's contractures, the scar tissue of hepatic cirrhosis and in the tissues around silicone breast implants as well as the granulating wound. The exact origin of myofibroblasts is uncertain, but is probably from the multi-potential cells around the capillaries. Radiation damage and cancer chemotherapy delay the onset of myofibroblast development and hence delay healing. The natural mechanism of contraction proceeds most rapidly if the wound is free from infection (Bendy, 1964), but is impeded by necrotic tissue, wound eschar of dead skin, and the application of a rigid wound dressing.

Epithelialisation

This is a mechanism whereby epidermal structures spread across the surface of an open wound. The epithelial defect is initially plugged by a fibrin coagulum and the epithelium turns downwards over the edge of the underlying dermis. At 24 hours large basal cells are mobilised on the undersurface of the dermis. By 48 hours the advancing epithelial edge has undergone cellular hypertrophy and mitosis. Epithelial cells respond to loss of contact by moving in response to that loss; thus migration ceases on meeting the opposite edge. The process involves not only migration of cells but cell mitosis and differentiation (Viaziam *et al.*, 1964).

As the epithelium grows across the wound surface there is minimal development of the rete pegs which usually interlock epidermis and dermis. Thus, wounds healing by epithelialisation are prone to loss of the epithelial layer by minimal trauma such as the removal of adhesive tape. The rate of epithelialisation may be enhanced by increased tissue oxygenation (Hunt and Pai, 1972) and maintaining a moist wound (Winter and Scales, 1963) and epidermal growth factor may accelerate wound repair (Buckley, 1985). Infection, the presence of necrotic tissue and excessive granulation tissue retard epithelial cover.

The natural healing processes often spontaneously heal wounds, so that a small, full-thickness wound in an elderly patient may heal with conservative treatment. However, the site of injury is also important as, for example, a large burn on the neck will result in immobility and distortion

Table 13.2 Factors delaying wound healing

General	Local
Age	Inadequate blood supply
Malnutrition	Haematoma formation
Cancer	Foreign-body implantation
Anaemia	Necrotic tissue
Systemic infection	Wound infection
Steroid treatment	Radiotherapy
Vitamin and trace metal deficiency	Recurrent trauma
Cancer chemotherapy	Duration of surgery
Diabetes	Experience of surgeon
Jaundice	Suture material
Uraemia	Wound tension
Obesity	
Hypothermia	
Anti-inflammatory drugs	
Sex	

with wound contraction, and, similarly, distortion after healing may result in loss of use in a hand.

The technical aspects of wound management are most important but general and local factors which may result in metabolic compromise of the healing process are also significant and are listed in Table 13.2. It is worthy of note that many of the factors which predispose tissue to breakdown (as discussed in Chapter 3) also delay wound healing.

Protein turnover reduces with age and quadriplegia (Claus-Walker *et al.*, 1982) and is reflected in a slower rate of healing, while in elderly patients there is an increased incidence of wound and anastomotic complications. This may be multifactorial with concomitant malnutrition, vitamin deficiences, co-existing neoplasia and its treatment (Smith, 1985) and a poor local blood supply. In addition, a brief pre-operative illness may profoundly affect wound healing (Goodson, 1987).

Hypoxia and ischaemia predispose to infection and, when established, the fibroblasts must compete with bacteria and inflammatory cells for oxygen and nutrients. Collagen synthesis is reduced and breakdown enhanced, thus collagen content of the wound is reduced. When coupled with cellular necrosis and the inability of collagen to grow, the breakdown of wound healing is inevitable. Uraemia (Yue, 1987) inhibits fibroblasts, while in jaundice fibroblast proliferation and the formation of new blood vessels are both delayed. Steroids depress the inflammatory response essential if wound healing is to proceed further with a similar absence of fibroblasts and new vessels. If steroids are started after the inflammatory phase of wound healing there is little effect on overall healing. Radiation causes cell death by damaging DNA, causing mutations and disrupting intracellular metabolism.

Severe protein calorie malnutrition has long been implicated in the failure of wounds to heal because of defective synthesis of both collagen and ground substance, while associated deficiencies of vitamins A, C and D impair healing and new bone formation and calcium, zinc, copper and manganese are essential minerals involved in healing (Hallams and Lasek, 1985).

THE MEASUREMENT OF WOUND HEALING

The precise measurement and management of secondary wound healing has been a major difficulty. The accurate measurement of healing in skin defects is fundamental both to their management and to study the rate and quality of healing. Biological surfaces are not flat, and direct contact between the instrument and the surface should be avoided to prevent contamination. The conventional method used to measure epithelial regrowth has been either to lay a sterile transparent sheet on the wound and then to trace the wound margins (Gowland-Hopkins and Jamieson, 1983) or to take a 35-mm colour slide photograph of the wound with a rule in the picture to provide a scale (Myers and Cherry, 1984). Direct tracing is simple and cheap but not acceptable because of damage or contamination of the wound, while simple photography suffers distortions because central projection does not have enough information to avoid scaling errors when measuring a surface curved in three dimensions. A stereophotogrammetric camera has been developed (Bulstrode *et al.*, 1986), linked to a metrograph and computer, which allows accurate, reproducible measurements of irregular defects in three dimensions. The accuracy and precision of this

Table 13.3 A comparison of stereophotogrammetry with the two systems currently in use – surface area. Accuracy and precision in per cent

Surface area (mm²)	Stereo photogrammetry		Direct tracing		Simple photography	
	Accuracy	*Precision*	*Accuracy*	*Precision*	*Accuracy*	*Precision*
10	0.9	2.2	60.0	75.0	43.0	80.0
50	0.6	1.8	29.0	40.0	23.0	26.0
140	0.6	2.1	16.5	21.0	10.7	17.0
405	0.9	2.1	10.0	18.0	16.0	17.0
790	0.8	1.8	5.8	12.0	8.6	34.0
1 200	1.1	1.8	0.3	10.5	3.9	11.5
2 050	1.0	1.9	3.7	8.6	1.6	11.0
3 260	1.0	2.0	5.8	10.2	4.0	11.0
4 540	0.7	2.2	4.0	6.2	3.2	12.0
6 380	0.7	1.7	2.9	6.7	5.1	11.1
9 840	0.6	1.8	0.4	4.9	10.0	10.3
14 110	0.8	1.8	2.3	5.7	8.5	10.7
Mean	0.81	1.9	11.7	18.2	11.4	21.0

Table 13.4   A comparison of stereophotogrammetry with the two systems currently in clinical use – area measurement of ulcers in patients. The 95 per cent confidence interval presented as percentage of mean

Surface area	Stereo photogrammetry	Direct tracing	Simple photography
8	5.5	48.0	45.7
12	3.8	37.8	19.6
15	4.3	60.3	47.7
16	5.9	19.0	9.1
16	1.9	64.6	66.0
82	2.7	29.0	21.6
92	3.1	57.0	36.0
114	2.0	17.6	11.0
125	1.8	21.6	14.1
134	2.6	23.4	15.9
Mean	3.36	37.8	28.6

system has been measured and compared with the two simpler methods (Table 13.3). The precision is better than 2 per cent and it is accurate to within 1 per cent for edge length and area in models of chronic leg ulcers whose dimensions were known and exactly measured under similar circumstances. Volume, the most difficult to measure, gives an accuracy of just over 5 per cent with a precision of under 2 per cent. With patients' ulcers the precision is 2 per cent for edge length and 3.4 per cent for area. These results are between 5 and 10 times better than direct tracing and simple photography (Table 13.4).

The accuracy with which an epithelial edge can be identified by the naked eye, a possible limiting factor, has been measured on fixed preparations or healing wounds on pigs. The mean error was found to be 240 μm, with a confidence limit of 440 μm. The rate of healing of chronic leg ulcers was then studied in clinical trials on patients. Stereophotogrammetry alone had errors consistently smaller than the changes being measured in the clinical trial, clearly indicating that it was the only system which can be used validly to study rates of healing in this model. It is also unique, in being able to non-invasively measure volume to within 5 per cent. This would prove of value in assessing the treatment of deep wounds, such as pressure sores.

Although the time to complete healing in granulating wounds is the only absolute value which can be used when studying the efficacy of different treatments for delayed wound healing (Svedman, 1983), it is expensive and time-consuming in resources and allows data to be collected only on those defects which heal within the period of observation. Using the stereogrammetry technique to compare the weekly measurements of edge length and surface area, and comparing these with the time taken to heal 30 patients each with an ulcer, it has been possible to describe the natural history of

Table 13.5 Prediction accuracy calculated from proportion of times to complete healing (TTCH) correctly predicted to the nearest week from each of the variables found to have a significant correlation with the actual TTCH

Variable measured	Proportion predicted to within one week (%)	Predictor factor
% change edge week 2	30	0.24
% change edge week 3	27	0.24
% change edge week 4	40	0.12
% change area week 3	47	0.11
% change area week 4	30	0.10

the healing of a chronic leg ulcer and to identify those factors which correlate with complete healing. In phase II of the healing process, that of rapid healing, the percentage change in surface area in week 3 was found to be a good predictor of time to complete healing (Table 13.5). If the value for week 3 was multiplied by a factor of 0.11 it was able to predict the total time to complete healing to within 1 week in half of the ulcers (Bulstrode *et al.*, 1987).

Further studies using the stereoscopic camera system have been carried out to study therapeutic measures which may influence healing rates of leg ulcers (Bulstrode *et al.*, 1988). Topical irrigation with normal saline has been shown to produce healing of chronic leg ulcers (Goode *et al.*, 1982). To further investigate this effect a randomised controlled trial was designed comparing the effect of topical amino acid solution irrigation of leg ulcers with normal saline. Exclusion criteria included a haemoglobin level of less than 10 g, active arthritis, diabetes, cardiac insufficiency, a peripheral vascular index of less than 0.9 or a diastolic blood pressure greater than 100 mmHg. The patient was then admitted to the trial following cleansing of the ulcer. The standard broad-spectrum amino acid solution produced a significantly higher rate of healing than normal saline. High osmolarity saline, however, produced significantly slower healing rates. Thus, in the first investigations of therapeutic management using the stereophotogrammetric system the application of amino acids does appear to enhance healing in chronic leg ulcers and it is an effect not dependent upon the osmolarity of the solution used.

The advent of this sophisticated measuring system for chronic skin defects may have provided new opportunities for studies in the management of delayed healing. Certainly, the accuracy of the system and its unique capacity to measure in three dimensions offers the prospect of the rationalisation of therapeutic measures to influence delayed cutaneous healing.

REFERENCES

Alexander, J. W. and Meakins, J. L. (1971). Natural defence mechanisms in clinical sepsis. *Journal of Surgical Research*, **11**, 148–161

Bendy, R. H. (1964). Relationship of quantitative wound bacterial counts to healing of decubitus. *Antimicrobial Agents and Chemotherapy*, **4**, 147–152

Buckley, A. (1985). Sustained release of epidermal growth factor accelerates wound repair. *Proceedings of the National Academy of Sciences*, **82**, 7340–7344

Bulstrode, C. J. K., Goode, A. W. and Scott, P. J. (1986). Stereophotogrammetry for measuring rates of cutaneous healing: a comparison with conventional techniques. *Clinical Science*, **71**, 437–443

Bulstrode, C. J. K., Goode, A. W. and Scott, P. J. (1987). Measurement and prediction of progress in delayed wound healing. *Journal of the Royal Society of Medicine*, **80**, 210–212

Bulstrode, C. J. K., Goode, A. W. and Scott, P. J. (1988). A prospective controlled trial of topical irrigation in the treatment of delayed cutaneous healing in human leg ulcers. *Clinical Science*, **75**, 637–640

Claus-Walker, J., Ferrante, N. D., Halstead, L. S. and Tavelia, D. (1982). Connective tissue turnover in quadriplegia. *American Journal of Physical Medicine*, **61**, 130–140

Cohen, I. K. and Keiser, H. R. (1976). Disruption of healed scars in scurvy: the result of disequilibrium in collagen metabolism. *Plastic and Reconstructive Surgery*, **57**, 213–215

Dunphy, J. E. and Udupa, K. N. (1955). Chemical and histochemical sequences in the normal healing of wounds. *New England Journal of Medicine*, **253**, 847–851

Gabbiani, G. (1971). Granulation tissue as a contractile organ: a study of structure and function. *Journal of Experimental Medicine*, **135**, 719–730

Goode, A. W., Wilson, I. A. I., Kirk, C. J. C. and Scott, P. J. (1982). Topical nutrition – a preliminary report. In Johnson, I. D. A. (ed.), *Advances in Clinical Nutrition*, MTP Press, Lancaster, pp. 339–349

Goodson, W. H. (1987). The influence of a brief pre-operative illness on post-operative healing. *Annals of Surgery*, **205**, 250–255

Gowland-Hopkins, N. F. and Jamieson, C. W. (1983). Antibiotic concentrations in the exudate of venous ulcers: the prediction of healing rate. *British Journal of Surgery*, **70**, 532–534

Grillo, H. C. (1964). Derivation of fibroblasts in the healing wound. *Archives of Surgery*, **88**, 218–224

Hallams, G. and Lasek, J. (1985). The effect of topical zinc absorption from wounds on growth and the wound healing processes in zinc-deficient rats. *Scandinavian Journal of Plastic and Reconstructive Surgery*, **19**, 119–122

Hunt, T. K. (1974). Diagnosis and treatment of wound failure. *Advances in Surgery*, **8**, 287–301

Hunt, T. K. and Pai, M. P. (1972). The effect of varying ambient oxygen tensions on wound metabolism and collagen synthesis. *Surgery, Gynaecology and Obstetrics*, **135**, 561–567

Kellerymyer, R. W. and Graham, R. C. (1968). Kinins: possible physiologic and pathological roles in man. *New England Journal of Medicine*, **279**, 754–759

Myers, M. B. and Cherry, G. (1970). Zinc and the healing of chronic leg ulcers. *American Journal of Surgery*, **120**, 77–81

Peacock, E. E. and van Winkle, E. (1972). *Wound Repair*. Second edn, Saunders, Philadelphia

Rudolph, R. (1980). Contraction and the control of contraction. *World Journal of Surgery*, **4**, 279–287

Smith, R. W. (1985). Effects of vinblastine, etoposide, cisplatin and bleomycin on rodent wound healing. *Surgery, Gynaecology and Obstetrics*, **161**, 323–326

Svedman, P. (1983). Irrigation of leg ulcers. *Lancet*, **ii**, 532–533

van Winkle, W. (1967). Wound contraction. *Surgery, Gynaecology and Obstetrics*, **125**, 131–142

van Winkle, W. (1968). The epithelium in wound healing. *Surgery, Gynaecology and Obstetrics*, **127**, 1089–1115

Viaziam, C. B., Matoltsky, A. G. and Mescow, H. (1964). Epithelialisation of small wounds. *Journal of Investigative Dermatology*, **43**, 499–506

Winter, G. D. and Scales, J. J. (1963). Effect of air drying and dressings on the surface of a wound. *Nature*, **197**, 91–92

Yue, D. K. (1987). Effects of experimental diabetes, uraemia and malnutrition on wound healing. *Diabetes*, **36**, 295–299

14

Biomechanics of Tissue Distortion and Stiffness by Magnetic Resonance Imaging

Steven I. Reger, Thomas F. McGovern and Kao Chi Chung

INTRODUCTION

Compression of soft tissues and their deformation under externally applied forces are the limiting factors in the fitting of body support systems in orthotics and prosthetics and wheelchair seating. Tissue pressure and strain are also important determinants of comfort on beds and mattresses. Measurement of muscle cross-sectional area can also be used to estimate contraction strength and function in ergonomics. Through the use of magnetic resonance imaging (MRI), a safe and non-invasive method for measuring tissue shapes *in vivo* has become available. By observing the response of atomic nuclei in magnetic fields, this technique can reconstruct longitudinal and transverse views of internal tissue structures from skin surface to bony prominences (Crooks, 1985). Without any known harmful effects, magnetic resonance techniques can provide clear views of anatomy and pathology of internal body structures in the gravity environment of recumbent human subjects.

The objective of this work was to determine the application of MRI techniques for measurement of soft tissue deformation *in vivo* on various support surfaces to aid in the design of cushions for wheelchair and seating use. These preliminary studies have produced significant information about the effect of externally applied pressure on the dimension changes of muscle, fat and skin and the compatibility of tissues and cushion for load transfer. The effect of normal loads on the skin causing transverse or tangential displacement of the subcutaneous muscle tissues was also demonstrated.

METHODS

MRI signals were generated, processed, stored and displayed initially by the Siemens 0.3 Tesla Magnetom System and later by Technicare 0.6 Tesla Teslacon Imaging System. The preliminary results reported here were

Table 14.1   Subject characteristics

Subject	Level of injury	Time since injury (years)	Body weight (kg)	Age (years)
Male paraplegic	L1	4	56	23
Male normal	n.a.	n.a.	64	23
Male paraplegic	T4	10[a]	70	25
Female paraplegic	T11	4	59	46
Female normal	n.a.	n.a.	61	38

[a] Daily electrical stimulation of gluteal tissues for nearly 1 year.

taken from 5 subjects, 3 males and 2 females. A summary of subject characteristics are shown in Table 14.1. The construction of the imaging systems restricted the subjects to lying supine in the tube, preventing the usual sitting posture from being studied. Supine subjects, supported on various cushions under the buttocks, could be studied for interface pressure and tissue deformation. One support arrangement allowed the buttocks to hang freely without cushion contact, while in another arrangement sand bag weights in increments up to 10 kg were used on the right iliac crest to increase loading of the tissues at the trochanter and the ischial tuberosity. Both bony areas are commonly involved in tissue breakdown.

The subjects were supported by 75 mm (3 inch) thick polyurethane foam cushions (E&J Durafoam or Scimedics Laminair). The interface pressure was measured under bony prominences before and after each imaging run by using the Scimedics pressure evaluating system (Talley Medical Ltd, Borehamwood) with a transducer bag of 6500 mm^2 effective surface area. The applied surface load was then calculated from the measured pressure and the transducer surface area. An imaging run was averaged from 4 samples requiring less than 10 minutes. Between runs the position of the subject was maintained constant by registering the location of surface anatomic landmarks on the support table. Images of the cross-sectional anatomy were scanned through the ischial tuberosity and the greater trochanter of the femur. Images were displayed on the CRT and hard copies made on photo negative films. Cursor control on the CRT display allowed measurement of tissue dimensions, cross-sectional areas and signal intensity in localised areas.

RESULTS

Observations

Clear images of the cross-sectional anatomy of the subjects were recorded by the signal acquisition and processing equipment, as previously described by Reger *et al.* (1986). Transverse views of the normal and paraplegic subjects are shown in Figures 14.1 and 14.2. These views were taken at the level of the greater trochanter and the ischial tuberosities of the supine subjects. Sharp contrast is evident between muscles and the subcutaneous fatty tissues. The bony prominences with surrounding bursa, gluteus muscles, fat and skin are clearly shown in the figures. The boundaries between subcutaneous fat and the skin are less well defined, owing to the poor contrast of the similar resonance signal and are often indistinguishable. Healthy, thick soft tissues are shown for a normal subject in Figure 14.1(A) in the free-hanging unsupported gluteal area. When supported on a foam cushion, not visible in Figure 14.1(B), the same tissues show reduction in thickness as a result of body weight and the external load applied anteriorly over the iliac crest on one side. The muscular tissues of the paraplegic subject shown in Figure 14.2(A) are poorly contrasted from the fatty tissues, possibly indicating the state of disuse atrophy. The extent of tissue atrophy is more clearly indicated by the increased reduction of tissue thickness upon loading of the paraplegic shown in Figure 14.2(B) from that of the normal, illustrated in Figure 14.1(B). Incremental loadings produced similar and proportional changes in both male and female subjects. Reduction of tissue tone in paraplegia is also indicated by the extensive lateral tissue bulge near the trochanter in Figure 14.2(B), suggesting increased coupling of vertical load to transverse elongation in the lateral tissues indicating tension and shear loading in that direction.

Measurements

To analyse changes in tissue dimensions under the applied loading, muscle thickness and the thickness of the skin and subcutaneous tissues were measured vertically from the bony prominence to the skin surface posteriorly at the support interface. The total tissue thickness from bone to skin surface was also plotted as a function of the mean interface pressure, which was measured at the interface before and after each imaging run, representing the different loading conditions from free hanging to body weight to added external weight loading. In some subjects the gluteus muscle width was also measured for each loading condition from the longest straight line across the muscle area in the lateral direction. In normal and paraplegic subjects of similar stature the cross-sectional area of the gluteus muscle was also measured from the images at the same loading levels. The muscle area of the normal was found to be nearly two times greater than the paraplegic muscle at any load level measured. Collectively these changes indicated significant differences in dimensions and load response between normally innervated and paraplegic tissues.

The tissue dimensions were plotted as a function of the measured surface

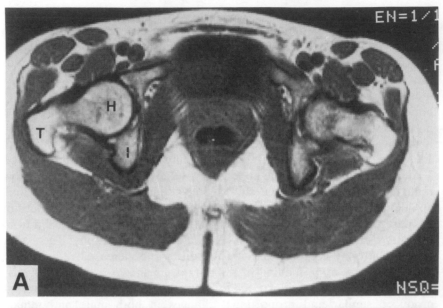

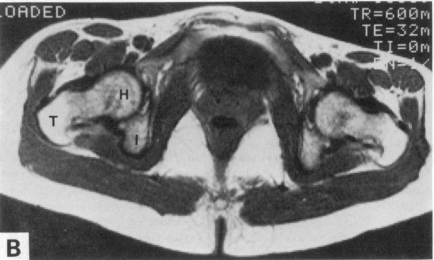

Figure 14.1 (A) Transverse magnetic resonance image of normal female near ischial tuberosities. Tissues without external support, free hanging. (B) Transverse magnetic resonance image of normal female near ischial tuberosities. Loaded tissues on the right side with flat cushion support below. T: trochanter of femur; H: head of femur; I: ischium

pressure for each load and location. The changes in total tissue thicknesses are shown for each bony prominence in Figure 14.3 for the male and in Figure 14.4 for the female subjects. In general, thicker tissues were

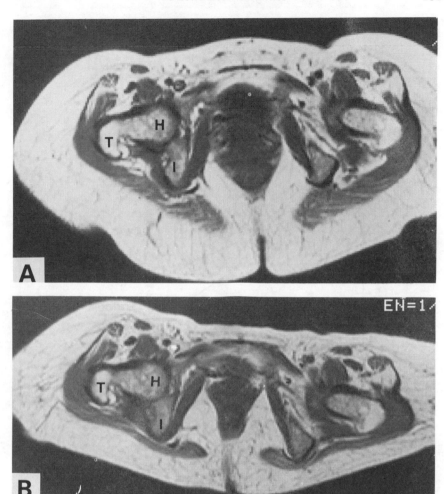

Figure 14.2 (A) Transverse magnetic resonance image of paraplegic female near ischial tuberosities. Tissues without external support, free hanging. (B) Transverse magnetic resonance image of paraplegic female near ischial tuberosities. Tissues loaded on the right side with flat cushion support below. Note blood vessel distortion by the mechanical environment. T: trochanter of femur; H: head of femur; I, ischium

observed in the normal subjects than in the paraplegics at any load, with the exception of the paraplegic female at zero load. Rapid reduction in tissue thickness was evident with increasing surface pressures for both normal and the denervated tissues. The paraplegic tissues were maximally compressed or indented and bottomed out under their own body weight at the bony prominences without additional weight. The additional external

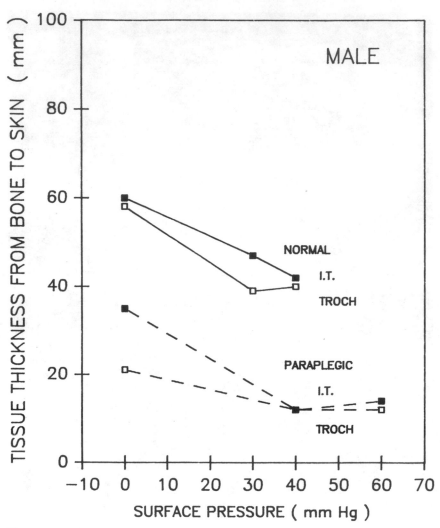

Figure 14.3 Reduction of tissue thickness with increasing surface pressure for male subjects

weight caused no further reduction of tissue thickness; it increased surface pressures only. On the normal tissues, however, the additional weight could cause further reduction of thickness at all locations except at the male trochanter.

Effects of Muscle Stimulation

One of the subjects, a long-term, high-level spastic paraplegic male, had

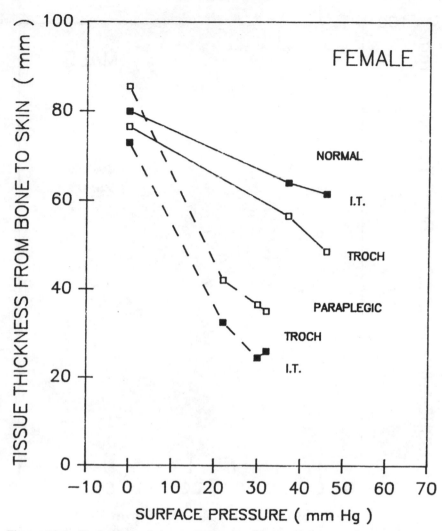

Figure 14.4 Reduction of tissue thickness with increasing surface pressure for female subjects

been undergoing daily functional electrical stimulation of the gluteal and quadriceps muscles bilaterally for nearly 1 year prior to the magnetic resonance imaging of this study. During this time, he reported remarkable increase in muscle bulk both anteriorly and posteriorly in his thighs. This reversal of his persistent muscle atrophy is evident in Figure 14.5, which shows his tissue thickness as a function of surface pressure. These curves at both the ischial tuberosity and the trochanter illustrate tissue characteristics intermediate between the paraplegic and normal. Initial tissue thickness and the slope of the curves from zero load to body weight are similar

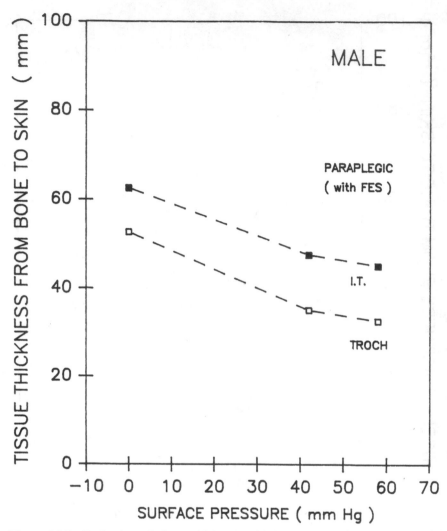

Figure 14.5 Reduction of tissue thickness with increasing surface pressure for paraplegic male subject after daily muscle stimulation for nearly one year

to normal tissue and do not bottom out with the added load. The decreasing slope at the higher loads, however, indicates abnormal response to load which is less than normal but not as reduced as the paraplegic. The suggested improvement in tissue stiffness towards the normal may be the benefit of induced muscle contractions during the pulsatile functional electrical stimulation.

Load Deformation Characteristics of Soft Tissues and Cushions

Materials used for body support may cause soft tissue trauma from incorrect load transfer at the tissue support interface. Despite the ubiquitous nature of this problem, no objective assessment of the support materials for individual need has been developed. The efficacy of the load transfer from the support cushion to the tissues is limited by the stiffness of the structures causing the load. For equal loads, a difference in stiffness

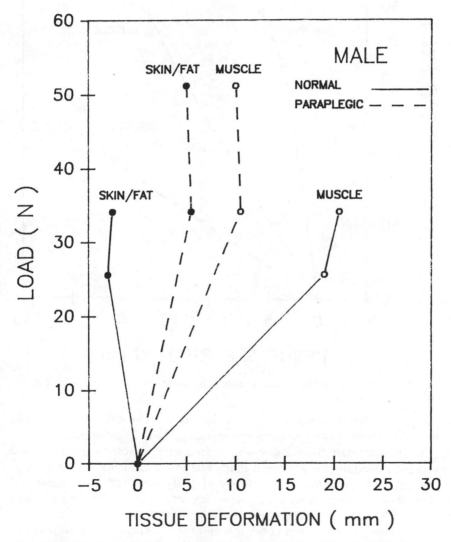

Figure 14.6 Load deformation curves for soft tissues in male subjects

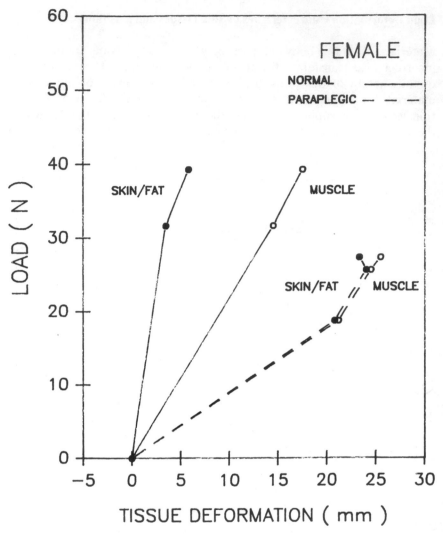

Figure 14.7 Load deformation curves for soft tissues in female subjects

results in higher deformation of the lower stiffness component, which leads to tangential or shear loads and hammocking at the tissue interface.

To further study the compressive deformation of soft tissues and foam support materials, the averaged individual tissue deformation under normal and added loads were calculated and compared with measured compressive characteristics of foam supports. Tissue deformation was calculated as the difference between thickness of each tissue type in the free-hanging, unsupported condition and the thickness of the same tissue in each loaded condition, measured vertically from the photographic MRI

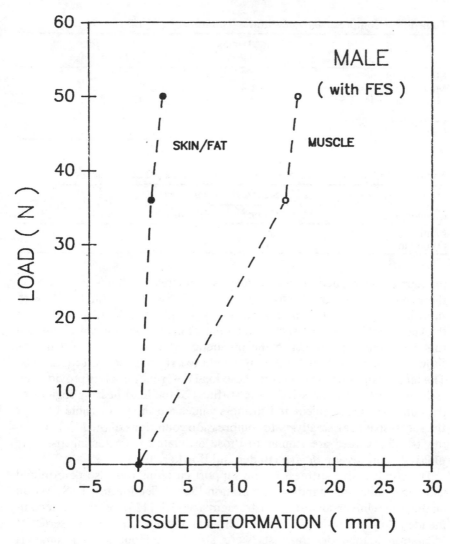

Figure 14.8 Load deformation curves for soft tissues in paraplegic male subject after daily muscle stimulation for nearly one year

data. This technique produced consistent resolution of the change in gluteal muscle thickness, whether the subjects were male or female, normal or paraplegic. The poor resolution between subcutaneous fat and skin produced uncertain thickness data for each, and thus the combined thickness of the two tissues was reported. The deformation of each tissue is plotted as the mean of two observations, one from the trochanteric and the other from the ischial area. The plots of deformation are shown in Figures 14.6 to 14.8 as functions of the applied load calculated from the measured

Table 14.2 Compressive tissue stiffness (N/mm)

	Average muscle	Average fat and skin
Male paraplegic	3.2	6.2
Male normal	1.4	−8.5
Male paraplegic FES	2.4	27.6
Female paraplegic	0.9	0.9
Female normal	2.2	9.0

Table 14.3 Compressive cushion stiffness (N/mm) (25 per cent deflection)

Cushion type	Indenter size (diameter)	
	203 mm	*70 mm*
Laminair	18.8	4.4
Durafoam	15.4	3.6

pressure. The reduction in thickness with increasing loads is shown on these plots as positive deformation for all tissues. Normal skin with subcutaneous fat in the male subject was found anomalously to increase thickness with increasing surface loading. This observation was attributed to subject motion artefact in the magnetic resonance image. All tissues showed changes in slope from body weight to externally loaded conditions. The initial slopes of the curves in these load deformation plots provided an estimate for the compressive tissue stiffness of the load-bearing regions of the buttocks. These calculated stiffness values are shown in Table 14.2 for the successive near-steady-state compression conditions of the MRI experiments. The values are similar to those estimated from testing tissue in uniaxial compression *in vivo* (Bader and Bowker, 1983).

The compressive stiffness of the support cushions was also determined using the industrial standard indentation load deflection test (ASTM) on an Instron Universal testing instrument (model 1123) using the recommended 203-mm (8-inch) diameter circular indenter. A second series of identation load deflection tests were also carried out using a smaller, 70-mm diameter circular indenter to simulate more anatomically sized loading and the local changes in the cushion characteristics. The tests were made in the compression mode and the load was measured at a specified cushion deflection under the indenters. The initial cushion thickness was measured after 4.5 N (1 lbf) was applied for 1 minute through the indenter. The indenter was then lowered into the cushion to 75 per cent of the initial height and held for 1 minute. This load, divided by the distance travelled, was used to calculate the compressive stiffness of the cushion. The compressive stiffness obtained with the 8-inch-diameter indenter is known in the industry as the ILD (indentation load deflection) value of the foam. As shown in Table 14.3, the values obtained with the smaller, 70-mm-diameter indenter approximated the tissue stiffness values closer than those obtained with the industrial standard 8-inch-diameter indenter. The results in Table 14.3 also show that the compressive cushion stiffness is dependent on the indenter size: a 2.9 times increase in diameter resulted in a 4.3 times increase of compressive stiffness of the cushion. As a result of this foam property ILD designations will overestimate cushion stiffness in low-deflection seating applications.

CONCLUSIONS

Soft-tissue deformations in vivo could be measured at high resolution using the convenient, safe and non-invasive method of magnetic resonance imaging. The transverse images of the soft tissues and bony prominences showed thicker tissues in normal subjects at every pressure, leading to the realisation that higher pressure gradients from skin to bone must exist in the paraplegic tissues than in the normal. Bottoming out of the paraplegic tissues showed the increased risk of tissue trauma caused by total compression and the resulting obstruction of blood flow. The border between subcutaneous fat and skin was not clearly defined, but normal muscle tissue yielded sharp margins with clear images with some exceptions. The average stiffness of the combination of skin and fat seems to be larger than the observed average stiffness of the muscle tissues.

The industrial standard 8-inch-diameter indenter proved too large for cushion measurement. Tested with the smaller indenter, the stiffness of the cushions showed more reasonable match to the paraplegic tissues particularly to muscles. The lateral 'bulging' and transverse distortion of the paraplegic tissues under vertical compressive loading indicated the need for precise matching of shape and material of the support surface to the tissue contours. The judicious use of contoured supports may preserve soft tissue padding under bony prominences and reduce pressure gradients by containment of tissues in the seating support. Functional electrical stimulation showed similar effect in reducing pressure gradients by the increase of muscle bulk and the increase of tissue thicknesses. The investigation of the effect of pulsating current on the stiffness properties of paraplegic tissues will continue.

REFERENCES

American Society for Testing and Materials: *Standard Methods of Testing Flexible Slab Urethane Foam*, ASTM:D1564-71
Bader, D. L. and Bowker, P. (1983). Mechanical characteristics of skin and underlying tissues in vivo. *Biomaterials*, **4**, 305–308

Crooks, L. E. (1985). An Introduction to Magnetic Resonance Imaging. *IEEE Engineering in Med. and Biol.*, **4**(3), 8–15

Reger, S. I., Chung, K. C. and Paling, M. (1986). Weightbearing tissue contour and deformation by magnetic resonance imaging. Proceedings of RESNA 9th Annual Conference, Minneapolis, RESNA, Washington DC, pp. 387–389

15

Effects of Compressive Loading Regimens on Tissue Viability

Dan L. Bader

INTRODUCTION

The peak pressures and the pressure gradients, present at the interface between the soft tissues and patient support, are considered to be one of the primary initiating factors in tissue breakdown. These interface pressures are transmitted through the soft tissues, establishing interstitial stresses and strains, which may be sufficient to impair the integrity of the local blood supply and lymphatic circulation. If the interface pressure is maintained then cell necrosis will follow, leading to tissue breakdown and the development of pressure sores. The mechanical nature of the soft tissues will undoubtedly influence the breakdown process. Hence, areas with minimal soft-tissue covering over bony prominences are more susceptible to breakdown than is an area with significant subcutaneous tissue and reduced mechanical stiffness.

The importance of time of loading has been shown in terms of tissue tolerance levels (Reswick and Rogers, 1976), and is particularly relevant to the immobile and insensitive subjects who are less inclined to relieve pressures. This makes them a prime target for pressure sore formation. One of the means of reducing the time of pressure application and hence relieving localised stresses that are potentially damaging to the soft tissues is by periodic shifting of position. This may be achieved for the debilitated subject by regular turning, although this is only possible if a care attendant is available. Some subject groups, for example the spinal-cord injured with satisfactory upper-body strength and co-ordination, practice regular lift-offs from the support surface in their wheelchair. Externally powered support surfaces can be designed to provide the pressure relief effect for the immobile subject. In particular, ripple mattresses, generally powered via an electric motor, have been routinely used to continually transfer body weight across the support areas.

The frequency of movement giving rise to pressure relief is an important factor, although this clearly will depend upon the recovery characteristics of the individual tissues. One report has suggested that wheelchair-bound paraplegics relieve their pressure every 30 minutes and that every 2 hours they should lie down for approximately 15 minutes (Griffith, 1963). Other investigators have recommended a time for continuous sitting of 20 minutes (Fisher and Patterson, 1983), although these authors found that one group of patients exceeded that time regularly with no apparent ill-effects. It is probable that an individual prescription of inter-lift-off interval for a given patient is required (Merbitz *et al.*, 1985).

Although pressure relief is undeniably advantageous, it should be mentioned that repetitive loading itself may also predispose to tissue trauma. In a series of studies it was found that repetitive mechanical loading (10 000 cycles a day over a 3-week period) to a rat's foot pad caused soft-tissue hypertrophy in normal rats and led to ulceration in neurectomized rats (Brand, 1976). Similar progressive destruction of muscle and later of skin has been proposed in a pig model (Daniel *et al.*, 1981).

There have been several attempts to indicate acceptable combinations of pressure and time in terms of tissue tolerance (Reswick and Rogers, 1976; Daniel *et al.*, 1981). Their results are indicated in Figure 16.1. However, these studies did not take into account the viability of the tissue, which is dependent upon an adequate supply of nutrients supplied by the blood. The measurement of blood flow to localised tissue areas is thus an essential part of the assessment of tissue viability.

A series of reports have described the effects of external loading on skin blood flow, using various techniques including radioisotope clearance (Daly *et al.*, 1976, Larsen *et al.*, 1979), photoplethysmography (Bennett *et al.*, 1984), and transcutaneous oxygen tension (Newson and Rolfe, 1982). The latter technique involves a small, surface-mounted, heated sensor under which local hyperaemia is induced, allowing measurements of the potential for oxygen delivery in relation to metabolic needs. It has been employed to objectively assess skin viability in various clinical conditions (Young *et al.*, 1981; Dowd *et al.*, 1983), and has been found to enable repeatable measurements to be made of the effects of load on tissue viability. An oxygen electrode was mounted in a flat indenter attached to skin surface. Loads were applied incrementally through the indenter for short periods of time until a cut-off load was reached with the transcutaneous oxygen tension (T_cPO_2) falling to zero. This is equivalent to the critical occlusion pressure. The tissue response for a group of both healthy young male subjects and elderly subjects was measured (Bader and Gant, 1985). Examination of an individual response yields information on the levels of pressure and time which the localised tissue areas may tolerate in terms of the oxygen levels available to the viable cells. The level of tolerable pressure was shown to vary considerably between individuals. However, the relationship between applied pressures and tissue oxygen level showed certain characteristic features, as illustrated in Figure 15.1.

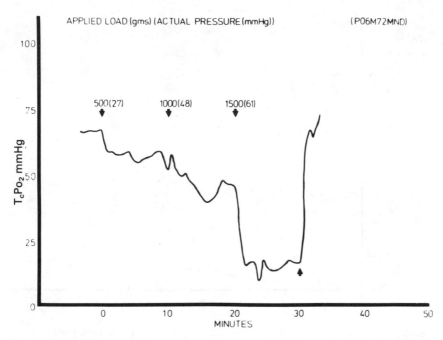

Figure 15.1 Changes in transcutaneous oxygen levels as a result of prolonged loading at the sacrum. Male subject, 72 years of age, with motor neurone disease

Firstly, for each period of constant loading there was some variation in T_cPO_2 levels about a mean value. These levels decreased gradually for initial applied pressures and then at an increasing rate as the applied pressure was increased. Finally, the T_cPO_2 recovered to the unloaded resting level following the removal of the load. It was clear that the clinician must restrict pressures at the sacrum of this subject to below 61 mmHg (8.1 kPa), if prolonged tissue ischaemia leading to cell necrosis is to be avoided.

EFFECTS OF PROLONGED LOADING

A recent publication detailed the response of a mixed group of 20 elderly subjects (mean age 61 years) to the application of prolonged external loads (Bader and Gant, 1988). In order to combine the data for all these patients, the results were presented in terms of relating applied pressure, for a prescribed period of time, to relative changes in transcutaneous oxygen tension, an approach previously recommended by Sacks *et al.* (1985). The results of each subject were estimated as a percentage reduction of the unloaded resting value of transcutaneous oxygen tension,

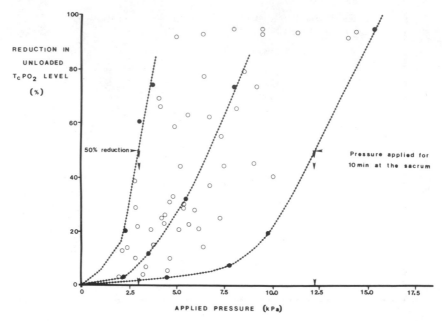

Figure 15.2 Composite plot showing the effects of applied pressure on trans-cutaneous oxygen tension at the sacrum. ● indicates data points for the three individuals whose responses are illustrated, ○ indicates data points for the remaining 17 subjects

at a known applied pressure (Figure 15.2). The form of the individual curves were distinctly biphasic, with an initial 'toe-in' section of variable length and gentle gradient followed by a linear region of increased gradient. In the first phase there is compression of the soft tissues and the integrity of the blood circulation is maintained. At higher pressures in the second phase the protection provided by the soft tissues is minimal and relatively small changes in applied pressure produce a significant reduction in T_cPO_2 levels. However, the results also demonstrated the considerable scatter and a wide range of applied pressures required to significantly reduce T_cPO_2 levels (Figure 15.2). For example, to achieve up to 50 per cent reduction of the unloaded value, applied pressures in the range of 22 mmHg (3.0 kPa) to 92 mmHg (12.2 kPa) were required. This response reflected both the diversity of clinical conditions within the subject group and intrinsic factors specific to the individual subject, such as the state of the local vascularity and nutrition.

Detailed examination of these results indicated no obvious trends with respect to age, sex and clinical condition. It was interesting, however, that the three subjects with a history of pressure sores attained arterial occlusion at relative low values of applied pressure, namely 40, 45 and 47 mmHg (5.3, 6.0 and 6.3 kPa). This may predispose these subjects to further tissue breakdown at the sacrum.

In these tests the recovery of the T_cPO_2 levels generally occurred within 1 minute of load removal. This recovery was evaluated after an applied pressure had been reached which had significantly reduced the T_cPO_2 levels. An extension of this work was to investigate the effects of repeated loading and recovery, to investigate its possible role in cumulative tissue breakdown.

EFFECTS OF REPEATED LOADING

The experimental system has been described in detail elsewhere (Bader and Gant, 1985, 1988). To review briefly, the system consists of a balanced beam with a movable weight at one end counterbalancing a loading pan

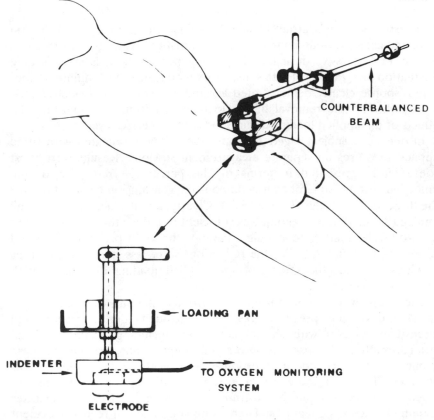

Figure 15.3 Experimental system to provide prolonged loading at the sacrum

directly above a rigid indenter (Figure 15.3). The indenter, incorporating a transcutaneous oxygen electrode (Radiometer model E5243), was attached to the flat surface of the sacrum using a double-sided adhesive ring. Stable thermal vasodilation was obtained after about 15 minutes. The tissues are loaded for a period of 10–15 minutes, with a moderate interface pressure of about 30 mmHg (4.0 kPa), followed by load removal for 2–5 minutes. The load is then reapplied and the cycle is repeated on two more occasions.

The corresponding pressures at the interface between the indenter and the sacrum were measured using one pneumatic cell of the Oxford pressure monitor (Bader and Hawken, 1986). The pressure was measured both before and after the main test procedure. This has been recently superseded by a doughnut pneumatic cell which has been designed to be attached to the base of the rigid indenter. This permits continuous monitoring of interface pressures during the loading and recovery phases.

Results

The response from a group of healthy subjects (age range 22–33 years) have indicated various consistent characteristics, typically illustrated in Figure 15.4. Firstly, during each loading period there is considerable fluctuation in T_cPO_2 level with some recovery during the 10-minute period. The response clearly demonstrated a rapid recovery to unloaded T_cPO_2 level following the removal of the loading conditions. In addition, the effects of the applied loading diminished with successive cycles.

In one male subject, aged 24 years, the test was repeated with three applied pressures on separate measurement sessions. Results were most conveniently presented in terms of the percentage reduction of the unloaded resting value of transcutaneous oxygen tension against time for the three loading cycles (Figure 15.5.). Clearly, an interface pressure of 62 mmHg (8.3 kPa) at the sacrum was sufficient to reduce the oxygen tension to zero levels on all three loading cycles. At the lower pressures of 48 and 55 mmHg (6.4 and 7.3 kPa) the reductions were less significant, and, as previously noted, the effects of the applied loading diminished with successive cycles.

These tests were also performed on a group of patients considered to be at risk of developing pressure sores. These included elderly, immobile and insensitive subjects with clinical conditions including traumatic spinal lesions, multiple sclerosis and lower-limb amputations. In some of these debilitated patients a normal response, as indicated in Figure 15.4, was obtained. However there was a group of patients whose response to repeated loading is typically illustrated in Figure 15.6. This demonstrates certain characteristic features. There is no suggestion of recovery evident during the initial loading cycle. Following load removal, the recovery

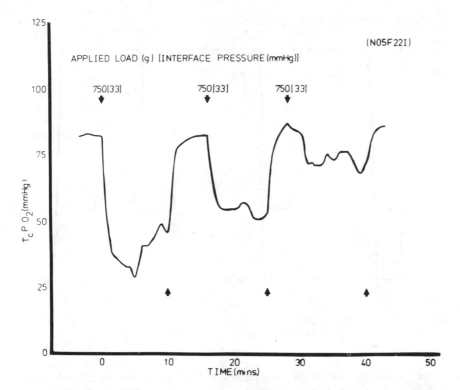

Figure 15.4 Changes in transcutaneous oxygen levels as a result of repetitive loading at the sacrum of a 21-year-old healthy male. An arrow pointing up indicates application of load; one pointing down indicates removal of load

period of 2 minutes was not sufficient for the T_cPO_2 levels to return to the initial resting value. Any subsequent loading appeared to have a cumulative effect by reducing the T_cPO_2 levels below those of the initial loading cycle.

DISCUSSION

The series of studies described in this chapter use the measurement technique for transcutaneous oxygen tension to monitor changes produced by the application of various loading regimes to localised areas of soft tissue. These measurements are performed with heated sensors as the absolute values of T_cPO_2 at physiological temperatures are small and any changes would have to be interpreted with caution. It is accepted that at the elevated temperatures normal blood flow regulation was abolished and the perfusion under the electrode was mainly determined by the arterial

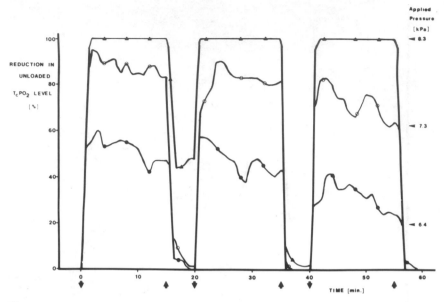

Figure 15.5   Effects of repetitive loading with three different applied loads on the transcutaneous oxygen tension at the sacrum

blood pressure. Although the absolute T_cPO_2 levels measured were undoubtedly elevated, it was the relative changes which were of interest, as interface pressures were increased up to the critical arterial occlusion pressure.

There were two distinct tissue responses produced as a result of cyclic loading. It is proposed that these responses may be explained in terms of tissue physiology. In one case (Figure 15.4), the recovery characteristics suggest a normal physiological reaction, as typified by reactive hyperaemia (see Chapter 12). Similar response has also recently been found with repetitive loading at the ischial tuberosity (Bader *et al.*, 1986). There is clearly an active vasomotor response mechanism, which produces a diminished effect on subsequent loading cycles. If the cycles were continued, the reduction in oxygen levels would presumably reach an asymptotic value. This response may be a direct result of the mechanical stresses which can transduce the release of biochemicals, such as histamine and prostaglandins, which are known vasodilators. The normal response may also be due partly to the anoxic state of the tissue during the loading phase. By comparison, the alternative response (Figure 15.6) is indicative of an impaired control mechanism. The time permitted for tissue recovery, namely 2 minutes, was inadequate and would inevitably lead to diminished oxygen levels on repeated loading and eventual tissue ischaemia. The recommended value of pressure relief every 20 minutes (Fisher and

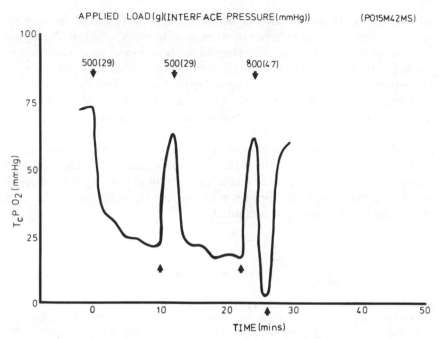

Figure 15.6 Changes in transcutaneous oxygen levels as a result of repetitive
loading at the sacrum of a 42-year-old male with multiple sclerosis

Patterson, 1983) is clearly inadequate for such a subject, who would
require more frequent and extended periods of pressure relief. This may
prove impossible by push-up alone even for the most athletic wheelchair
user, who would thus require additional help from a care attendant or from
externally powered pressure-relieving supports.

The previous investigation showed little correlation between tissue
response and clinical condition (Bader and Gant, 1988). This has also been
suggested in the present study, as subjects with the same clinical condition,
for example those with multiple sclerosis or the spinal-cord injured,
demonstrated one or other of the distinct reponses to cyclic loading. This
supports the clinical observation that within the spinal-cord-injured
population some subjects are significantly more prone to the development
of pressure sores than others (Sacks *et al.*, 1986). This emphasises the
importance of intrinsic factors in determining susceptible subgroups of
patients. Further studies involving the physiological control mechanisms of
the microcirculation, particularly in the state of tissue ischaemia, are
required. Such an approach was followed in a study on an elderly group of
in-patients and demonstrated an impairment in the ability to increase
blood flow following localised stimulation (Ek *et al.*, 1984). The authors
postulated that this was due to a decreased vascularisation in the papillae.
This is common in the ageing process, where the skin becomes thinner

(Ryan, 1973). However, this is believed to be a result of inadequate stimulus, since atrophic skin can be stimulated to vascularisation during the process of wound healing. Differences in skin blood flow response to loading may lead to identification of those patients who are most susceptible to pressure sore development upon hospital admission. This would lead to a redistribution of nursing care in a manner that would diminish the incidence and, necessarily, the overall cost of treatment. The use of a clinical rating evaluation, such as the Norton scale, can identify those generally at risk. Such subjects should be included in an extended study. Further work to investigate the effect of a variety of cyclic loading regimes is required. This should include an increased ratio of loading to recovery to simulate those clinical situations where patients do not adhere to a strict movement regime when not reminded.

REFERENCES

Bader, D. L. and Gant, C. A. (1985). Effects of prolonged loading on tissue oxygen levels. In Spence, V. A. and Sheldon, C. D. (eds), *Practical Aspects of Skin Blood Flow Measurements, Biological Engineering Society*, London, pp. 82–85

Bader, D. L. and Gant, C. A. (1988). Changes in transcutaneous oxygen tension as a result of prolonged pressures at the sacrum. *Clin. Phys. Physiol. Meas.*, **9**, 33–40

Bader, D. L. and Hawken, M. B. (1986). Pressure distribution under the ischium of normal subjects. *J. Biomed. Eng.*, **8**, 353–357

Bader, D. L., Evans, R. and Beavis, A. (1986). The effects of repeated loading on tissue viability. *Oxford Orthopaedic Engineering Centre Annual Report* No. 13, pp. 49–51

Bennett, L., Kavner, D., Lee, B. Y., Trainor, F. S. and Lewis, J. M. (1984). Skin stress and blood flow in sitting paraplegic patients. *Arch. Phys. Med. Rehabil.*, **65**, 186–190

Brand, P. W. (1976). Pressure sores – the problem. In Kenedi, R. M., Cowden, J. M. and Scales, J. T. (eds), *Bedsore Biomechanics*, Macmillan Press, London and Basingstoke, pp. 19–23

Daly, C. H., Chimoskey, J. E., Holloway, G. A. and Kennedy, D. (1976). The effect of pressure loading on the blood flow rate in the human skin. In Kenedi, R. M., Cowden, J. M. and Scales, J. T. (eds), *Bedsore Biomechanics*, Macmillan Press, London, pp. 69–77

Daniel, R. K., Priest, D. L. and Wheatley, D. D. (1981). Etiological factors in pressure sores: an experimental model. *Arch. Phys. Med. Rehabil.*, **62**, 492–498

Dowd, G. E., Linge, K. and Bentley, G. (1983). The effect of age and sex on normal volunteers upon the transcutaneous oxygen tension in the lower limb. *Clin. Phys. Physiol. Meas.*, **4**, 65–68

Ek, A.-C., Lewis, D. H., Zetterqvist, H. and Svensson, P.-G. (1984). Skin blood flow in an area at risk for pressure sore. *Scan. J. Rehab. Med.*, **16**, 85–89

Fisher, S. V. and Patterson, P. (1983). Long-term pressure recordings under the ischial tuberosities of tetraplegics. *Paraplegia*, **21**, 99–106

Griffith, B. H. (1963). Advances in the treatment of decubitus ulcers. *Surg. Clinic. N. America*, **43**, 245–260

Larsen, B., Holstein, P. and Lassen, N. A. (1979). On the pathogenesis of pressure sores. Skin blood flow cessation by external pressure on the back. *Scand. J. Plas. Reconstr. Surg.*, **13**, 347–350

Merbitz, C. T., King, R. B., Bleiberg, J. and Grip, J. C. (1985). Wheelchair push-ups: measuring pressure relief frequency. *Arch. Phys. Med. Rehabil.*, **66**, 433–438

Newson, T. P. and Rolfe, P. (1982). Skin surface PO_2 and blood flow measurements over the ischial tuberosity. *Arch. Phys. Med. Rehabil.*, **63**, 553–556

Reswick, J. B. and Rogers, J. E. (1976). Experience at Rancho Los Amigos Hospital with devices and techniques to prevent pressure sores. In Kenedi, R. M., Cowden, J. M. and Scales, J. T. (eds), *Bedsore Biomechanics*, Macmillan Press, London and Basingstoke, pp. 301–310

Ryan, T. J. (1973). Structure pattern and shape of the blood vessels of the skin. In Jarrett, A. (ed.), *The Physiology and Pathophysiology of the Skin*, Academic Press, London, pp. 577–651

Sacks, A. H., O'Neil, H. and Perkash, I. (1985). Skin blood flow changes and tissue deformations produced by cylindrical indentors. *J. Rehab. Res. Dev.*, **22**, 1–6

Sacks, A. H., Perkash, I. and O'Neil, H. (1986). Skin deformation and blood flow under external loading. *V. A. Rehabilitation R & D Progress Reports*, pp. 97–98

Young, K. C., Railton, R., Harrower, A. D. *et al.* (1981). Transcutaneous oxygen tension measurements as a method of assessing peripheral vascular disease. *Clin. Phys. Physiol. Meas.*, **2**, 147–151

16

Effects of Mechanical Stresses on Lymph and Interstitial Fluid Flows

Narender P. Reddy

INTRODUCTION

Viability of soft tissue subject to external mechanical stresses is important from the standpoint of pressure sore formation. Pressure sores, also known as decubitus ulcers, develop as a result of prolonged excessive mechanical stresses on tissue.

During sitting or reclining for extended periods of time, normal individuals relieve stresses that are potentially damaging to their tissues by periodic shifting of position. Patients with loss of sensation, such as those with spinal-cord injuries, do not sense or relieve these excessive stresses. The type and magnitude of stresses generated in the tissue depend on body build and the types of cushion used to support the body (Garfin *et al.*, 1980; Garber and Krouskop, 1982; Garber *et al.*, 1982; Reddy *et al.*, 1982). Garfin and co-workers (1980) observed large areas of high pressure generated in human subjects lying prone and supine on beds of various types. In certain regions, pressure up to 200 mmHg (26.7 kPa) was observed. In seated subjects the pressure beneath the ischial tuberosities exceeded well over 150 mmHg (20 kPa) (Kosiak *et al.*, 1958).

Although it is known that prolonged excessive stresses on tissue cause ulceration, the mechanisms of decubitus ulceration and associated damage processes are not clearly understood. Several investigators have produced pressure sores experimentally, in various animal species, by application of excessive and prolonged loads on skin and subcutaneous tissue. There is general agreement that an inverse relationship exists between the intensity and duration of load application required to produce ulceration (Figure 16.1). High external pressure requires only a short duration of loading, whereas lower pressure requires longer application times to cause equivalent tissue damage. There is a delay of 3 to 5 days between load application and external appearance of an ulcer at the skin surface.

The first systematic study of decubitus ulcer formation was attempted by Kosiak (1959), who applied external pressure of different intensities for various durations over dog femoral trochanter and ischial tuberosity. After release of pressure, he observed oedema and cellular infiltration immediately, which persisted for 1 or 2 days. Kosiak found an inverse relationship between pressure intensity and the application duration necessary to cause ulceration in dogs and rats. Ulceration generally appeared 3 or 4 days after the application of pressure. Since the intensities of applied pressure were larger than the intracapillary pressure, Kosiak advanced the hypothesis that ischaemia and capillary damage are the major factors leading to pressure-induced ulcers. Lindan (1961) found similar oedema and haemorrhage in rabbits after the release of external compression with pressure clips. In swine, Dinsdale (1974) observed an inverse relationship between the pressure intensity and loading duration necessary to produce ulceration experimentally. Daniel and Wheatley (1981) experimentally produced decubitus ulcers in swine using a computer-controlled electromechanical load applicator device. They also observed an inverse relationship between the critical pressure intensity and the duration necessary to cause ulceration (Figure 16.1).

Reswick and Rogers (1976) monitored the skin-cushion interface pressures on 800 volunteer normal human subjects and patients, and also found an inverse relationship between the intensity and duration of interface pressure which skin and subcutaneous tissues could tolerate (Figure 16.1). They provided a threshold curve separating acceptable and unacceptable combinations of pressure intensity and duration. Since then their curve has been used as a guideline for soft-tissue management in various seating clinics.

In all of the animal experiments discussed above, oedema persisted for at least 1 day after pressure release. These observations led the investigators to believe that ischaemia associated with blood vessel occlusion is the major factor in decubitus ulcer formation. Very few attempted to study transport processes. Persistent oedema and cellular infiltration indicate definite disturbances in the transport mechanism.

Prolonged hypoxia ultimately leads to ulceration; but the precise damage mechanisms are not well understood. Also, the phenomenological models postulated by the early investigators do not explain the observed intensity–duration effects. Holloway and associates (1976) found that skin blood flow ceases when the external pressure reaches mean arterial pressure. If oxygen is the only factor, all pressure intensities in excess of the capillary closing pressure should produce ulceration in the same duration of time.

We believe that prolonged excessive mechanical stresses may cause breakdown of skin and subcutaneous tissue, by impairing microcirculation, lymph circulation, and interstitial transport process. The purpose of this chapter is to examine the effects of mechanical stresses on lymphatic and interstitial fluid circulation.

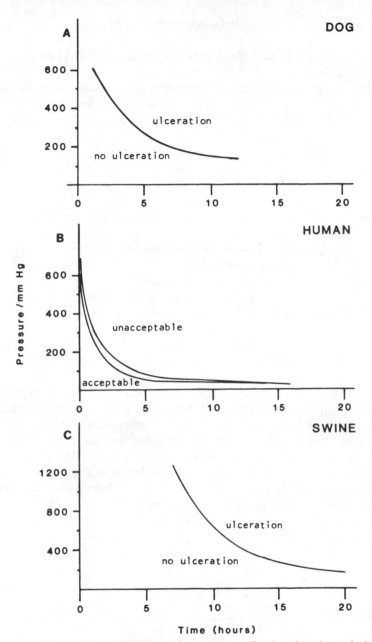

Figure 16.1 Threshold pressure intensity versus application duration relationship for the following conditions. (A) Ulceration observed in experimental dogs. (From M. Kosiak, 1961. Reproduced by kind permission of *Arch. Phys. Med. Rehab.*) (B) Acceptable interface pressures in human subjects. (From J. B. Reswick and J. E. Rogers, *Rancho Los Amigos Hospital Technical Report*, submitted to Social and Rehabilitation Service, 1976.) The two curves represent different humidity conditions at the buttock–cushion interface. (C) Experimental production of ulcers in swine. (From Daniel and Wheatley, 1981. Reproduced by kind permission of *Arch. Phys. Med. Rehab.*)

PHYSIOLOGY OF THE LYMPHATIC SYSTEM

The lymphatic system is essentially a drainage system within the human body. It consists of a complex network of vessels and presents a major route for the transport of excess fluid, protein, and metabolic waste products from the tissue of origin into the blood circulatory system (Reddy 1986). Lymphatics are vessels and lymph is the fluid within the lymphatic system. Lymph from most parts of the body enters the blood circulatory system at the junction of the left subclavian and jugular veins via the thoracic duct. There are numerous valves along the lymphatic vessel network which aid in unidirectional motion of lymph from the periphery towards the jugular vein.

The interstitial fluid pressure is normally 2 to 4 mmHg (0.3 to 0.5 kPa) below the atmospheric pressure (Reddy *et al.*, 1981a). On the other hand, the jugular venous pressure is of the order of 4 to 10 mmHg (0.5 to 1.3 kPa) above the atmospheric pressure. Lymph is first absorbed by the terminal lymphatics and then propelled by the contracting lymphatics.

The Terminal Lymphatics

The terminal ramifications of the lymphatic system, the network of lymphatic capillaries which absorb lymph from the interstitial spaces, are collectively referred to as the terminal lymphatics. Unlike the larger lymphatics and collecting ducts, the terminal lymphatic vessels are made up of a single layer of endothelial cells (Figure 16.2). The lymphatic capillaries are 5 to 10 times more distensible than the blood capillaries (Nisimaru, 1982). Normally, the terminal lymphatics have flattened or uneven contours, varying in diameter from 1×10^{-5} to 6×10^{-5} m.

In most tissues, the overlapping inter-endothelial cellular junctions act as valves and allow unidirectional motion of interstitial fluid into the lumen of the terminal lymphatic (Figure 16.2). There is bulk flow of fluid, macro-

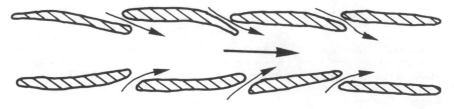

Figure 16.2 The interendothelial junctions of the terminal lymphatic (lymph capillary) act as valves and allow only undirectional motion of fluid from the interstitial spaces of the lumen of the terminal lymphatic

molecules and other substances into the lumen of the terminal lymphatic through these inter-endothelial junctions.

The inter-endothelial junctions are open whenever the pressure in the terminal lymphatics becomes smaller than the interstitial fluid pressure and are closed when the terminal lymphatic pressure exceeds the interstitial fluid pressure (Reddy, 1986; Reddy *et al.*, 1975a; Adair and Guyton, 1985). Leak (1980) and Casley-Smith (1976) believe that these junctions are rather large 'open' junctions several microns in width.

In normal conditions, only a small fraction of the endothelial junctions are open. As the interstitial fluid pressure starts increasing, an increasing number of junctions opens up. Thus the permeability of the terminal lymphatics is regulated by the fluid in the interstitial spaces.

The terminal lymphatics are held open by anchoring filaments (Figure 16.3). Electron microscopy has revealed that anchoring filaments are attached to the walls of the terminal lymphatics on one end and to the elastic tissue matrix (collagen fibres) on the other end (Leak and Burke, 1968). These anchoring filaments are like non-linear springs. During oedema (increased interstitial fluid volume), the inter-fibre distance between the collagen fibres increases owing to the matrix swelling. This would cause the anchoring filaments to apply a pulling force on the terminal lymphatic vessel walls (Reddy and Patel, 1989). Thus, in situa-

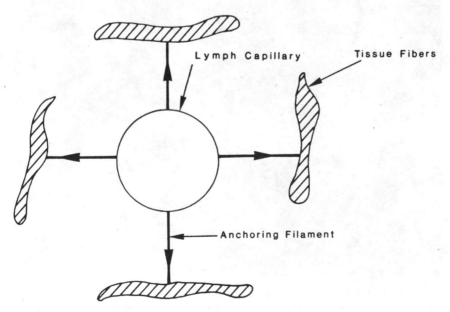

Figure 16.3   Diagramatic representation of the anchoring filaments in relation to the tissue fibre matrix and the terminal lymphatic

tions of increased interstitial fluid pressure, the anchoring filaments keep the terminal lymphatic from collapsing.

Lymph Propulsion Along the Contractile Lymphatics

Lymph propulsion along the lymphatic network is governed by certain extrinsic and intrinsic forces. The extrinsic forces are due to the movement of skeletal muscle and of various organs. The intrinsic forces are due to active contractions of smooth muscle on the walls of the lymphatics (Figure 16.4).

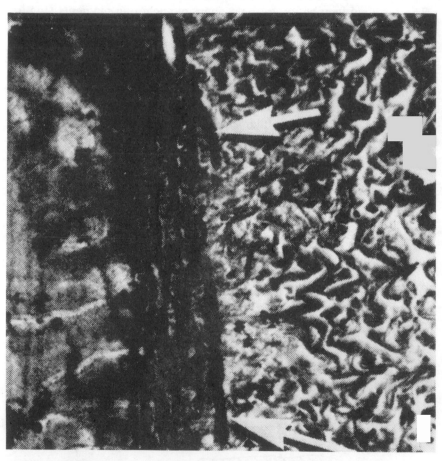

Figure 16.4 Wall of the thoracic duct (large lymphatic duct) contains several layers of smooth muscle cells (arrows); magnification ×80 (5 micron paraffin, modified crossman stain). (From Reddy and Staub, 1981. Reproduced by kind permission of Academic Press)

The intrinsic smooth-muscle contractions of the lymphatic vessels are regulated by three major factors: (1) the transmural vessel distention, (2) humoral mediators and (3) neural mediators. Lymphangion, the segment between two valves, contracts as a whole and is the basic functional unit of the lymphatic system. Distension of the lymphangion in the radial direction, or the wall hoop strain, is a stimulus for initiating the contractions. A contraction is initiated only if the stretch in the wall exceeds certain threshold value characteristics for each vessel segment (Mislin, 1971). Each contraction lasts for a given period of time followed by a period of relaxation. The contraction–relaxation cycles are myogenically controlled and are modulated by a number of humoral mediators. During the relaxation cycle the smooth muscle becomes refractory to further stimulation. During this refractory period, a contraction cannot be initiated even if the stretch of the wall exceeds the threshold value.

Characteristics of these contractions have certain similarity to those of the heart. The contraction cycle can be characterised into a diastolic phase and a systolic phase. The duration of the diastole depends on the upstream boundary conditions, which can be traced back to the interstitial fluid pressure. Duration of the systole, on the other hand, is an intrinsic factor and is a characteristic of the vessel. Similarly, the refractory period is a characteristic of the vessel. Both the contractile duration and the refractory period can probably be altered by humoral mediators.

Contractile activity usually starts in lymphangions adjacent to the terminal lymphatics and spreads progressively from one lymphangion to

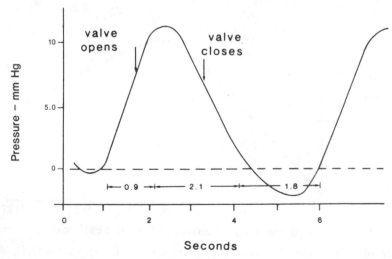

Figure 16.5 Details of representative pressure tracing in collecting lymphatic of rat mesentry. (From Zweifach and Prather, 1975. Reproduced by kind permission of *Am. J. Physiol.*)

the next, towards the thoracic duct (Reddy, 1974; Reddy *et al.*, 1975b, 1977). Contraction–relaxation cycles occur between 2 and 30 minutes, with an average 2–4-second contraction cycle (Zweifach and Prather 1975). The contraction phase is usually short (0.8–1.0 second), while the relaxation phase develops more gradually (Figure 16.5). The amplitude of pulsations and the base line pressure increase from segment to segment and increase with increasing vessel size.

Distension-induced Enhancement of Contractility

The lymphatic smooth muscle is sensitive to transmural pressure-induced wall stretch. The intensity of a contraction depends to a large extent on the amount of preload or the amount of hoop strain present in the wall just before the onset of the contraction; it increases with increasing initial vessel distension up to a point and then decreases with further increase in the preload (Figure 16.6). This relationship is similar to the Frank–Starling law of the heart in that the end diastolic stretch increases the strength of the next contraction. The distension-induced enhancement of contractility presents a physiological mechanism for self-regulation of the lymphatic pump; so as to pump more vigorously during increased demand. Also, this mechanism would allow smooth propagation of contractions from one segment to the next.

We have studied the regulation of motility in the largest lymph duct, the

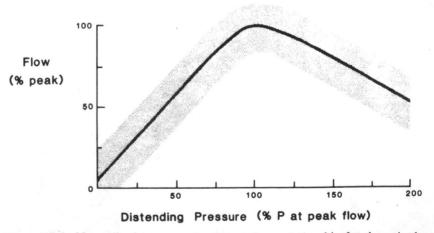

Figure 16.6 Normalised transmural pressure–flow relationship for thoracic duct perfused in anaesthetised ventilated dog. Solid line represents the best-fit polynomial. The shaded areas are ±1 s.e.m. (From Reddy and Staub, 1981. Reproduced by kind permission of *Microvasc. Res.*)

thoracic duct perfused in the anaesthetised dog (Reddy and Staub, 1981). After cannulating both ends of the duct, with chest open and ventilation constant, we perfused it with Krebs–Henselite with inflow and outflow pressure kept at the same level such that there was no net driving pressure gradient. Without any pressure gradient, flow through duct must be due to intrinsic smooth-muscle contractions. When we increased the transmural distending pressure (increased P_{in} and P_{out} simultaneously), the flow increased, as the distending pressure increased to certain level, and then declined (Figure 16.6). Our results, in a living animal, confirmed the earlier hypotheses (Reddy, 1974) and results *in vivo* using isolated vessels and vessel segments (McHale and Roddie, 1976).

Regulating Action of Biochemical Mediators

Several . biochemical mediators have a regulating effect on the lymph propulsion. The lymphatic smooth-muscle contractions can be modulated by a number of humoral mediators such as histamine, adrenaline, noradrenaline, 5-hydroxytryptamine (5-HT, or serotonin), prostaglandins (PGE_1, PGE_2, PGH, PGF_2, PGI), dopamine, acetylcholine (ACh), phentolamine, isoproterenol, ATP and ADP.

We have developed an experimental animal model for studying the effects of humoral mediators on lymphatic smooth-muscle contractions, in intact animals, using cannulated thoracic duct perfused in anaesthetised ventilated open-chest dogs (Reddy and Staub, 1981). With this model, the test substances can be either mixed in the perfusion fluid or administered intravenously. The advantage of the constant intravenous infusion of test substances into intact animals is that the agents reach the lymphatic vessel via the vasa-vasorum. The administration of the test substances through the vasa-vasorum simulates the physiological conditions more closely.

Catecholamines, in physiological concentrations, enhance the intensity of lymphatic contractions. Ohhashi *et al*. (1978) found dose-dependent increase in amplitude of contractions, in isolated longitudinal strips of bovine mesenteric lymphatics, with noradrenaline (10^{-6} to 10^{-5} M). Mawhinney and Roddie (1973) observed that norepinephrine (5–25 ng/ml) markedly increases contraction frequency in isolated bovine mesenteric lymphatic vessels. Our results (Reddy and Staub, 1981), using perfused thoracic duct in anaesthetised dogs, confirmed all these earlier findings with respect to the effect of catecolamines. We found 52 per cent and 134 per cent enhancement of perfused fluid flow rate, respectively, to intravenous infusion of epinephrine at 2×10^{-10} and 4×10^{-10} kg/(kg min). At 2×10^{-10} kg/(kg min), norepinephrine enhanced flow by 72 per cent.

Basal nervous activity does not appear to exist in the lymphatics because phentolamine, an α-blocker, did not decrease control lymph flow in our experiments (Reddy and Staub, 1981). The contractile response to transmural distending pressure appears to be mainly myogenic, since McHale and Roddie (1976) found that tetradotoxin, which blocks intramural nerve plexus, did not affect intrinsic contractility in isolated lymphatics.

5-hydroxytryptamine (5-HT), or serotonin, is an important vasoactive agent also known to increase intestinal motility. In our experiments, in perfused thoracic duct in intact dogs, 5-HT inhibited lymph flow. At intravenous infusion rates of less than 2×10^{-8} kg/(kg min), 5-HT had little or no effect on liquid pumping by the thoracic duct. At high infusion rates of 4×10^{-8} kg/(kg min), 5-HT had a biphasic effect. The flow rate increased transiently, but in most dogs it decreased to about half the control flow rate. In addition, 5-HT decreased flow when it was perfused through the lumen of the thoracic duct in concentrations of 10^{-6} to 10^{-5} M. Also, in our study, 5-HT increased resistance to flow under a fixed non-zero driving pressure gradient. All this evidence suggests that 5-HT contracts lymphatic smooth muscle, but the contraction takes the form of spasm and inhibits lymph propulsion.

Histamine is another important and well-known vasoactive agent. We observed that histamine infused intravenously at 1×10^{-9} to 4×10^{-9} kg/(kg min) consistently depressed the liquid pumping by the thoracic duct perfused in intact dogs.

Prostaglandins are important modulators of vascular smooth muscle contractions and play an important role in the control of blood pressure and flow. Prostaglandins E_1, E_2 and I_2 are potent vaso-dilators and inhibit lymphatic motility. In our thoracic duct perfusion experiments in intact dogs (Reddy and Staub, 1981), we found that intravenous infusion of PGE_1 decreased thoracic duct pumping in a dose-related manner (12–40 per cent inhibition at 1×10^{-9} to 4×10^{-9} kg/(kg min)). PGE and PGF are considered primarily local hormones which produce their effects upon cells in the vicinity of their site of release, since they are inactivated in the lung before reaching the arterial circulation. In spite of this, PGE_1 inhibited lymph propulsion in our study. Johnston *et al.* (1983) found that PGE_1 and PGE_2 in concentrations of 10^{-5} M inhibited contractions in isolated circular segments of bovine lymphatics. Ohhashi *et al.* (1978) tested several prostaglandins and found that both PGE_2 and PGI_2 caused dose-related reductions in amplitude of contractions.

Calcium ions are probably important for the control of pacemaking and for the propagation of impulse. Spontaneously active vessels are very sensitive to the calcium concentration (McHale and Allen, 1984).

EFFECTS OF MECHANICAL STRESSES ON REGIONAL LYMPH FLOW

Mechanical stresses can cause direct mechanical damage to the lymphatic system or could induce indirect damage by causing hypoxia in the tissue.

Lymph propulsion greatly depends on lymphatic smooth-muscle contractions. This smooth-muscle motility is highly sensitive to intravascular distention and circulating humoral mediators. Significant hypoxia can develop in the tissue as a result of external pressure application. This hypoxia, if prolonged, may damage lymphatic smooth muscle since smooth-muscle function is sensitive to anoxia. Prolonged occlusion of the lymphatic vessel, together with prolonged anoxia, can cause permanent damage to myogenic contractile mechanisms. Damaged smooth muscle or non-functional myogenic contractile mechanism causes impairment of lymph flow. Humoral mediators released during hypoxia, such as serotonin, histamine and prostaglandins, may further inhibit lymphatic smooth-muscle activity (Figure 16.7).

Anchoring filaments of the terminal lymphatics hold these vessels open during oedema. These filaments are delicate and can be easily damaged.

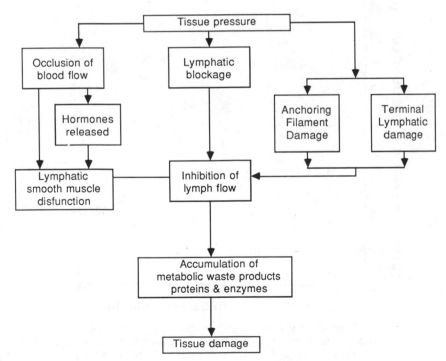

Figure 16.7 Hypothesis on the role of lymphatics in decubitus ulcer formation

External mechanical forces when prolonged could lead to permanent deformation in these filaments. Also, dislocation of the filaments could occur. With non-functional or dislocated anchoring filaments, terminal lymphatics would simply collapse during oedema, which then would lead to further build-up of metabolic waste products in the tissue.

Structural integrity of the delicate terminal lymphatics can be damaged more readily than the blood capillaries during external mechanical force application. Also, the inter-endothelial junctions could get damaged leading to impaired lymph absorption by the terminal lymphatics.

Impaired lymph flow may lead to accumulation of metabolic waste products, which in turn leads to the onset of tissue necrosis. Results of Miller and Seale (1981) support this hypothesis. They injected colloidal sulphur tagged with radioactive technitium[99] into the subcutaneous tissue in upper thighs of hind limbs of dogs and measured the radioactivity during

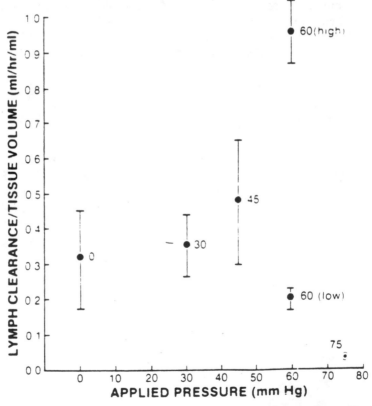

Figure 16.8 Tissue clearance of Tc-99m during external pressure application in experimental dogs. At 60 mmHg (8 kPa), high-clearance and low-clearance groups were noted. (From Miller and Seale, 1981. Reproduced by kind permission of *Lymphology*)

external compression with a dead-weight cylindrical device. They measured radioactivity in the tissue (through an external solid-state detector) at the injection site (loaded region) and also at the regional lymph node. Technitium accumulated at the lymph node and they therefore assumed that lymphatics cleared the tracer. Lymphatics cleared the interstitial fluid until external pressure reached 60–70 mmHg (8–9.3 kPa) and then lymph flow reduced to zero with further increase in external pressure (Figure 16.8).

EFFECT OF MECHANICAL STRESSES ON INTERSTITIAL FLUID FLUX

With application of external load, tissue deforms as the result of the response of the connective tissue matrix. Some blood vessels are immediately occluded, while others are occluded within the next few minutes as the load is transferred to deeper strata. Blood flow in a loaded region reaches a steady state in a time period of minutes (Daly *et al.*, 1976). In addition, there is a slow viscous flow of interstitial fluid and ground substance out of the region under pressure. The characteristic time for ground substance flow is of the order of a few hours (Kenyon, 1979). During indentation experiments on skin and subcutaneous tissues in anaesthetised pigs (Cochran *et al.*, 1980), we observed a continual increase of the indentation depth during the creep phase even after 6 hours of constant load.

We examined the effects of external pressure on interstitial fluid dynamics using a simple mathematical model (Reddy *et al.*, 1981b). Our theoretical analysis of interstitial dynamics suggests that the flow of interstitial fluid and ground substance plays a role in ulcer formation. Consider a circular cylindrical slice of tissue of radius a with pressure applied at the top surface (Figure 16.9). For simplicity, let the interstitial fluid pressure in this pressurised region, P_a, be uniform over the entire volume of the cylinder. Now consider a surrounding concentric cylindrical slice of tissue of radius R from the centre of the pressurised region. The rate of interstitial fluid flow from the region per unit length of the cylinder is proportional to the gradient in fluid pressure from the loaded region to the surrounding region. Also, the law of conservation of mass requires that the decrease of interstitial fluid volume in the pressurised cylinder is equal to the increase of interstitial fluid volume in or surrounding unloaded tissue. From these relationships, for a given ratio of initial volume to final volume within this central pressurised region, with prescribed parameters of porosity and fluid conductivity, the product of the loading duration t and the interstitial fluid pressure gradient between the pressurised region and

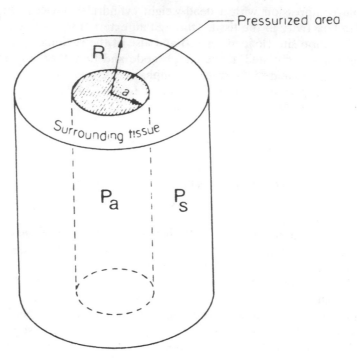

Figure 16.9 Tissue model for interstitial fluid flux calculations: inner cylinder tissue slice (radius a) of high interstitial fluid pressure surrounded by concentric tissue ring of low interstitial fluid pressure

the surrounding region $(P_a - P_s)$ equals a constant:

$$(P_a - P_s)t = \text{constant}.$$

If pressure in the surrounding region is negligible, then the product of pressure in the central region and loading duration is a constant. For example, if $(P_a - P_s)$ is 150 mmHg (20 kPa), we calculated that the time required for the interstitial volume to reach half its initial volume is approximately 1.8 hours. Thus it appears that there is an inverse relationship between pressure intensity and load duration required for the interstitial fluid volume to reach a given portion of its initial volume. This relationship is similar to the threshold intensity and duration relationship in external pressure experimentally observed in studies of ulceration.

The similarity between pressure–duration relationships in experimental production of ulceration and interstitial fluid flow suggests that slow viscous flow of interstitial fluid and ground substance may play a significant role in the mechanisms responsible for observed threshold pressure–time relationships, and therefore for tissue breakdown.

Although our simple, linear model predicts that interstitial fluid volume

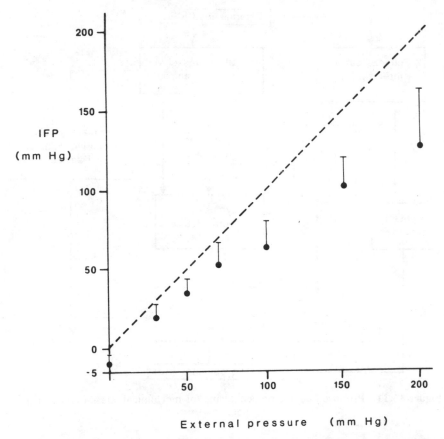

Figure 16.10 The relationship between external pressure and subcutaneous interstitial fluid pressure observed in the fore limbs of anaesthetised Yorkshire pigs. (Reddy *et al.*, 1981*a*. Reproduced by permission of *Am. J. Physiol.*)

approaches zero as time tends to infinity, it approaches a finite non-zero value and cannot be reduced indefinitely with time. More complex models are necessary for accurate prediction. However, the relationships between interstitial fluid pressure and stresses in solid tissue have to be taken into account.

As noted earlier, soft tissue contains networks of elastic elements, namely collagen and elastin, which are interspersed with blood and lymphatic capillaries and interstitial fluid. In healthy individuals, stresses distribute themselves so that the collagen network supports a substantial fraction of the load and protects the microvasculature from pressure-induced damage. Only a fraction of the externally applied load is transmitted to the interstitial fluid (Figure 16.10; Reddy, *et al.*, 1981*a*). However, in spinal-cord-injured patients, collagen in the soft tissue may be catabolised

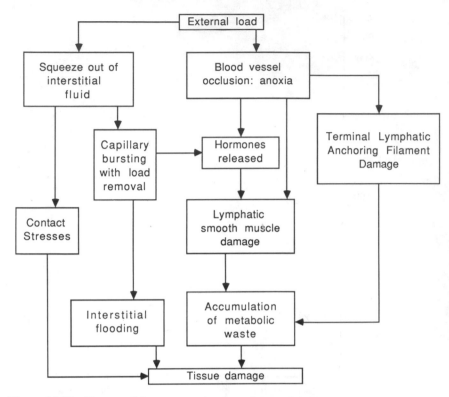

Figure 16.11   Proposed damage mechanisms for mechanical stress-induced tissue
necrosis

(Claus-Walker, *et al.*, 1982), leading to increased loading on the microvasculature, lymphatics, interstitial fluid, and ground substance. Thus spinal-
cord-injured patients might be more susceptible to decubitus ulcers (Bennett *et al.*, 1981).

   The following damage mechanisms are proposed (Figure 16.11). When
interstitial fluid is squeezed out of a tissue region, direct contact of the cells
induces contact stresses. These stresses on the fibroblasts cause rupture or
perhaps interrupt collagen synthesis by contact inhibition. This inhibition
and collagen breakdown continue even after the actual load is removed.
After squeezing out the interstitial fluid and load release, interstitial fluid
pressure becomes small (negative) enough to cause cavitation and capillary
bursting in the area previously affected by external load. Dinsdale (1974)
found increased vacuoles in cells after prolonged loading. This occurs
because the characteristic time for interstitial fluid flow is long compared
with the characteristic time for blood flow. Interstitial flooding and
subsequent protein transfer into the surrounding tissues takes place. At
this point, any loss of function in the lymphatics due to prolonged pressure

and hypoxia in smooth muscle also contributes to the process of tissue necrosis.

Soft tissue consists of several components: namely, the microvasculature, lymphatics, interstitial fluids, ground substance, cells, fibrous network and nerves. Very little is known about the responses of the lymphatic system and interstitial fluid to external pressure application at present. Also, further studies on skin microcirculation during prolonged loading are needed. The normal functioning of all major tissue components is probably essential for maintenance of tissue viability. Thus the study of mechanical stresses on skin and subcutaneous tissue presents a fruitful domain for microcirculatory and biomechanical research.

REFERENCES

Adair, T. H. and Guyton, A. C. (1985). In Johnston, M. G. (ed.), *Experimental Biology of the Lymphatic Circulation*, Elsevier, New York, pp. 13–44

Bennett, L., Kavner, D., Lee, B. Y., Trainor, F. S. and Lewis, J. M. (1981). Skin blood flow in seated geriatric patients. *Arch. Phys. Med. Rehab.*, **52**, 392–398

Casley-Smith, J. R. (1976). Functioning and interrelationships of blood capillaries and lymphatics. *Experentia*, **32**, 1–4

Cochran, G. V. B., Reddy, N. P., Brunski, J. B. and Palmieri, V. (1980). In *Proceedings of International Conference on Rehabilitation Engineering*, held in Toronto, Canada, June 13–18, 1980, pp. 163–166

Claus-Walker, J., DiFerrante, N., Halstead, L. S. and Tavella, D. (1982). Connective tissue turnover in quadriplagia. *Am. J. Phys. Med. Rehab.*, **61**, 130–140

Daly, C. H., Chimoskey, J. E., Holloway, G. A. and Kenedy, D. (1976). In Kennedi, R. M., Cowden, J. M. and Scales, J. T. (eds), *Bedsore Biomechanics*, University Park Press, Baltimore, Md, pp. 69–78

Daniel, R. K. and Wheatley, D. C. (1981). Etiologic factors in production pressure sores: experimental model. *Arch. Phys. Med. Rehabil.*, **62**, 492–498

Dinsdale, S. (1974). *Mechanical Factors in the Pathogenesis of Ischemic Skin Ulcers in Swine*, Ph.D. Thesis, University of Minnesota

Garber, S. L. and Krouskop, T. A. (1982). Body build and its relationship to pressure distribution in a seated wheelchair patient. *Arch. Phys. Med. Rehab.*, **63**, 17–20

Garber, S. L., Campion, L. J. and Krouskop, T. A. (1982). Trochianteric pressure in spinal cord injury, *Arch. Phys. Med. Rehab.*, **63**, 549–552

Garfin, S. R., Pye, S. A., Hargens, A. S. and Akeson, W. H. (1980). Surface pressure distribution of the human body in recumbent position. *Arch. Phys. Med. Rehab.*, **61**, 409–413

Holloway, G. A., Daly, C. H., Kennedy, D. and Chimosky, J. (1976). Effects of external pressure loading on human skin blood flow measurements. *J. Appl. Physiol.*, **40**, 597–600

Johnston, M. G., Kanelac, A. and Gordon, G. (1983). Effects of arachidonic acid and its cyclo-oxygenase and lypogenase products on lymphatic vessel contractility. *Prostaglandins*, **25**, 85–104

Kenyon, D. (1979). A mathematical model of waterflux through aortic tissue. *Bull. Math. Biol.*, **40**, 62–69

Kosiak, M. (1959). Etiology and pathophysiology of decubitis ulcers. *Arch. Phys. Med. Rehab.*, **40**, 62–69

Kosiak, M., Kubicek, W. G., Olson, M., Danz, J. N. and Kottke, F. J. (1958). Evaluation of pressure as a factor in the production of ischial ulcers. *Arch. Phys. Med. Rehab.*, **39**, 623–629

Leak, L. V. (1980). Lymphatic removal of fluids and particles in the mammalian lung. *Environ. Health. Persp.*, **35**, 55–78

Leak, L. V. and Burke, J. F. (1968). Ultrastructural studies on the lymphatic anchoring filaments. *J. Cell Biol.*, **36**, 129–162

Lindan, O. (1961). Etiology of decubitus ulcers; an experimental study. *Arch. Phys. Med. Rehab.*, **42**, 774–783

Mawhinney, H. J. D. and Roddie, I. C. (1973). Spontaneous activity in isolated bovine mesenteric lymphatics. *J. Physiol.*, **229**, 339–350

McHale, N. G. and Allen, J. M. (1984). Electrophysiological examination of neuromuscular transmission in bovine mesenteric lymphatics. *Irish J. Med.*, **153**, 220–232

McHale, N. G. and Roddie, I. C. (1976). The effect of transmural pressure on pumping activity in isolated bovine lymphatic vessels. *J. Physiol.*, **341**, 517–533

Miller, G. E. and Seale, J. (1981). Lymphatic clearance during compressive loading. *Lymphology*, **14**, 161–166

Mislin, H. (1971). Die kontraktilen eigenschaften der lymphagefasse. *Angiologica*, **8**, 79–85

Nisimaru, Y. (1982). Summary of our studies concerning the structure and function of lymphatic system. *Hiroshima J. Med. Sci.*, **31**, 145–192

Ohhashi, T., Kawai, Y. and Azuma, T. (1978). The response of lymphatic smooth muscle to vasoactive substances. *Pflugers Arch.*, **375**, 183–198

Reddy, N. P. (1974). *A Discrete Model of the Lymphatic System*, Ph.D. dissertation, Texas A & M University

Reddy, N. P. (1986). Lymph circulation: physiology, pharmacology and biomechanics. *CRC Critical Rev. Biomedical Engineering*, **14**, 45–91

Reddy, N. P. and Patel, K. (1989). Computer simulation of flow through the terminal lymphatics (in preparation).

Reddy, N. P. and Staub, N. C. (1981). Intrinsic propulsive activity of thoracic duct perfused in anaesthetized dogs. *Microvasc. Res.*, **21**, 183–192

Reddy, N. P., Krouskop, T. A. and Newell, P. H. (1975a). Biomechanics of a lymphatic vessel. *Blood Vessels*, **12**, 265–278

Reddy, N. P., Krouskop, T. A. and Newell, P. H. (1975b). A note on the mechanisms of flow through the terminal lymphatics. *Microvasc. Res.*, **10**, 214–217

Reddy, N. P., Krouskop, T. A. and Newell, P. H. (1977). A computer model of the lymphatic system. *Comp. Biol. Med.*, **7**, 181–197

Reddy, N. P., Palmieri, V. and Cochran, G. V. B. (1981a). Subcutaneous interstitial fluid pressure during external tissue loading. *Amer. J. Physiol.*, **240**, R327–R329

Reddy, N. P., Cochran, G. V. B. and Krouskop, T. A. (1981b). Interstitial fluid flow as a factor in decubitus ulcer formation. *J. Biomech.*, **14**, 879–881

Reddy, N. P., Patel, H., Cochran, G. V. B. and Brunski, J. B. (1982). Model experiments to study the stress distribution in seated buttock. *J. Biomech.*, **15**, 493–504

Reswick, J. B. and Rogers, J. E. (1976). In Kenedi, R. M. and Cowden, J. M. (eds), *Bedsore Biomechanics*, University Park Press, Baltimore pp. 301–310

Zweifach, B. W. and Prather, J. W. (1975). Micromanipulation of pressure in terminal lymphatics in the mesentery. *Am. J. Physiol.*, **228**, 1326–1351

Part IV
Technological Systems
for Patient Monitoring

17

Ischial Pressure Distribution Under the Seated Person

Dan L. Bader and M. B. Hawken

INTRODUCTION

One area in which technology may assist in the prevention of pressure sores is in the monitoring of physical conditions at the interface between the body tissues and a support surface. This is particularly relevant in the immobile and debilitated subject, who is especially prone to tissue breakdown. The extrinsic factors generally considered to be of importance in the assessment of tissue viability include normal pressure, shear stress, temperature, movement and moisture levels. This has led to the development of several non-invasive systems which measure accurately the pressure distribution at the patient–support interface (Garber *et al.*, 1978; Bader *et al.*, 1985). Clearly, tissue ischaemia will result if localised interstitial stresses reach values in excess of the capillary pressure, reported as 32 mmHg (4.3 kPa) by Landis (1930). However, as a result of the intervening soft-tissue layer, the level of tolerable pressure at the tissue interface will be generally higher, although its absolute value will depend upon the many intrinsic factors specific to an individual.

Support cushions should provide a safe, stable and comfortable means of transmitting loads to the body. The emphasis of much current design and research is on safety and on the reduction of the incidence of tissue damage in patients who are particularly at risk (Jay, 1983). This may be achieved in most cases by a support surface which provides a uniform pressure distribution over a maximal support area. It may, however, be necessary to reduce or remove pressure in particularly sensitive areas, and it must be possible to shape the support cushion accordingly with appropriate cutouts in the support surface. In addition to achieving clinically acceptable interface pressures, the choice of support cushion should be made with regard to other physical, functional and aesthetic factors (Ferguson-Pell *et al.*, 1986). These include stability, durability and temperature dissipation.

A support cushion is usually supplied to a disabled person in conjunction with a separate or integral cover. This cover is used primarily to minimise wear and soiling of the load-distributing element (Denne, 1981). For example, some foams are liable to deteriorate when subjected to repeated shear loading incorporating tensile stresses, unless they are adequately

223

covered by two-way stretch materials. Covered cushions are also cosmetically acceptable to the user and the removable covers facilitate regular cleaning. Ideally the cover should also be smooth, strong, flexible, durable, porous and absorbent. This additional layer of material interposed between the soft tissue and the cushion material will affect the pressure distribution at the tissue–support interface, and although covered cushions are in common use very little is known about the effects of cover materials on pressure distribution.

Previous Studies

There are several studies in which the distribution of pressure at the seating interface has been investigated (examples include Garber and Krouskop, 1982; Ferguson-Pell *et al.*, 1986; Engel, 1988). In one of these studies, 70 patients, each with a prior history of decubitus ulcers, were tested in a standard wheelchair on 4 different cushioning materials (Garber and Krouskop, 1982). The tissue pressure distribution was found to depend to a considerable extent on body build and weight. For any particular cushion, the responses of the subjects varied considerably, and individual subjects responded in different ways to the test cushions.

Engel (1988) reported that the presence of support cushions on a standard wheelchair with seat canvas reduced maximum pressures at the sitting interface by up to 50 per cent. In addition, the contents of the cushions filled with foam, gel, air and also viscoelastic foam were observed to move as the body moved, resulting in a fairly uniform pressure distribution.

An initial study using the Oxford pressure monitoring system investigated the pressure distribution at the ischium of a small group of normal subjects (Bader and Hawken, 1986). In order to make an objective evaluation of the support cushions, three pressure parameters were chosen. These included mean, maximum pressures and maximum pressure gradient, the latter indicating the extent of localised tissue distortion, in particular local shear strains, which have an important effect on the viability of tissues (Chow and Odell, 1974; Scales, 1982). Maximum pressure gradients of between 1.31 and 1.64 mmHg/mm (0.17 and 0.22 kPa/mm) were recorded.

The main finding of this study was that while the pressure distribution varied little if the subject sat still for up to a maximum of 15 minutes, if the subject stood up and then sat down again there was a significant variation in the measured pressure distribution. The authors attributed this variation to the postural changes produced by repositioning, which was later confirmed using a back shape measuring system (Riley and Bader, 1988). This inherent variation must be taken into account if a comparison between several different support surfaces is to be performed. The authors recommended that several sets of readings must be taken for each support surface and between each set of readings the subject should stand up and then sit down again. Thus variability due to repositioning will exist both within and between groups, and statistical methods will detect any extra variability due to differences between support surfaces.

Many types of cushions are available to the potential user, differing both in material and method of construction (Jay, 1983). Some commercially available cushions have been studied (Krouskop *et al.*, 1986), but the wide variety has so far precluded a comprehensive study of all current types. Of particular interest to many of those involved in UK seating clinics are those cushions which are widely supplied through the Disablement Services Authority. These include two foam cushions of different densities and several commercially available cushions which may be supplied to those subjects who are particularly susceptible to pressure sores and are generally unable to change their position when sitting (Cochrane and Wilshere, 1988).

This chapter discusses the investigation of the effects of these foam and gel cushions on pressure distribution at the ischium of a group of normal subjects. The investigation also included an assessment of the effects of various covering materials used with the two types of foam cushion.

THE PERFORMANCE OF SELECTED SUPPORT CUSHIONS

The experimental equipment used was identical to that described in the previous paper (Bader and Hawken, 1986). To review briefly, an adjustable seating system was used to maintain the subject in a standardised position. The flexible matrix of the pressure-monitoring system was attached centrally over the right ischium of each subject. The test procedure involved the subject sitting on each cushion while one complete scan of the pressure matrix was obtained, taking approximately 60 seconds. The subject then stood up for a sufficient time to allow the cushion to recover to its original thickness, before being repositioned on the cushion. The procedure was repeated a total of 5 times for each cushion. Cushions were presented in a random order for each subject. All pressure readings were transferred in digital form to a microcomputer (British Broadcasting Corporation, model B) and stored on disk for subsequent analysis. The position of a subject in the assessment chair is illustrated in Figure 17.1.

The 6 different support cushions used in the main study are described in Table 17.1. The cushions tested are all in regular clinical use, and the 3 gel cushions are available commercially. In addition, the rigid plywood support provided a useful assessment of ischial pressure distribution on a surface which was non-deformable at the load levels under investigation.

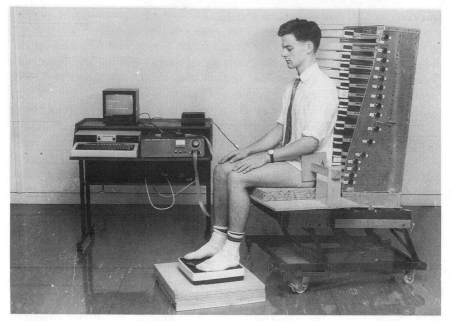

Figure 17.1   Test subject seated in standardised position on the assessment chair

Ten healthy male and 10 healthy female subjects were tested. The males had a mean age of 30 years (range 27–35) and a mean weight of 77 kg (range 63–91 kg) and the females a mean age of 25 years (range 19–33) and a mean weight of 58 kg (range 51–65 kg). The subjects were divided into body build types, thin, average, and obese, based on height, weight, sex and age. Using the same criteria as in a previous study (Garber and Krouskop, 1982), an average subject was defined as weighing between 90 per cent and 110 per cent of his or her ideal weight. Consequently, 17 of the total subjects were classified as being of average body build. Of the remainder, 2 (1 male, 1 female) were classed as thin and one female as obese.

The effects of covering materials were tested in a supplementary study. Cushions were made from each of the two foam bases previously studied (2 and 3 in Table 17.1). The cushion covering arrangements tested with each foam were: no cover at all; stockinette; two-way stretch terry-towelling; tweed; and a standard Department of Health PVC laminated cover (Ambla, Wardle Storey, Colne).

Ten healthy male volunteers were included in the study of covering materials. Their mean age was 29 years (range 20–44), and mean weight 72 kg (range 58–86 kg). Seven of these subjects were classified as being of average build and 3 were classed as thin. Five of the male subjects were included in both studies.

Table 17.1   Details of support cushions

Number	Description of support cushion
1	PVC-covered combination foam–gel cushion, 75 mm thick.
2	Medium-density polyurethane (PU) chip foam[a] cushion, 75 mm thick.
3	Composite foam cushion, 50 mm low-density PU foam[b] layer on top of 25 mm medium-density PU chip foam layer, 75 mm thick in total.
4	Medium-density PU chip foam cushion, 50 mm thick.
5	Gel cushion with pile fabric cover, 50 mm thick.
6	Vinyl-covered gel cushion with air cell surround.
7	Plywood surface.

[a] Medium-density (80–88 kg/m^3) reconstituted chip foam: indentation hardness to BS 3667 60–75 kg.
[b] Low-density (27–30 kg/m^3) foam: indentation hardness to BS 3667 16–20 kg.

Mechanical Testing of Cushions

The mechanical properties of 5 of the support cushions were tested in compression in a mechanical testing machine (Instron model 1122) at a crosshead speed of 5 mm per minute. Loads were applied with an indenter of spherical profile, approximating to the body contour in the ischial area. The radius of the spherical surface was 100 mm, and the overall diameter of the indenter was 150 mm. The maximum load applied to the indenter was 250 N, equivalent to a mean pressure of 14.1 kPa (106 mmHg). The composite nature of cushion 6 (Table 17.1) precluded the use of this localised mechanical test method.

Data Analysis

After the various parameters had been extracted, the arithmetic mean of each set of 5 parameter values was calculated. Thus for each parameter there were 6 values (1 for each cushion) for each of the subjects. Testing for homogeneity indicated that the variances of the pressure readings did not meet the assumptions required for parametric tests (Bader and Hawken, 1986). In consequence, the Friedman two-way analysis of variance was used in this study to test the hypothesis that there was no consistent difference between support cushions over the 20 subjects. A separate analysis was carried out for each pressure parameter. In the event of a significant result, the Wilcoxon critical range method (Colquhoun, 1971) was used to carry out unplanned comparisons between the cushions.

   Data from the tests of cushion covering material was also analysed by non-parametric methods, a separate analysis being performed for each pressure parameter. A 5-way data table was established, which contained the differences between pressure parameter values for the 2 foams for each of the covering materials. The differences were then ranked. The null hypothesis was that there was no interaction between foam and covering material, and therefore no systematic difference between the rank difference scores for the covers. A Friedman 2-way analysis was carried out to test this.

Results

A summary of the combined results from all 20 subjects is displayed in Figure 17.2. The Friedman analysis revealed a significant difference between cushions for each parameter at the 0.1 per cent level (Table 17.2). In considering each subject, it was possible to rank the support cushions in order of increasing value of pressure parameter. This order was not the same for each subject, and the Wilcoxon critical range test only showed a small number of statistically significant differences between cushions (Table 17.3). The most consistent differences were shown to exist between

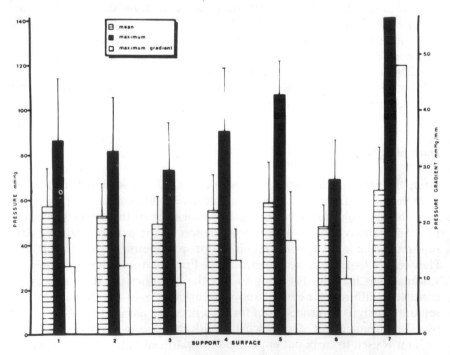

Figure 17.2 Summary of results for pressure parameters on the seven support surfaces, averaged for the twenty test subjects. ± Standard deviation indicated for all except support surface 7 (see text)

Table 17.2   Results of a Friedman analysis on 6 support cushions for all 20 subjects

Parameters of pressure distribution	*Support cushion* 1	2	3	4	5	6
A Mean mmHg	91	65.5	44.5	82	97	40
	(5)	(3)	(2)	(4)	(6)	(1)
B Maximum mmHg	84	66	37.5	88	111	33.5
	(4)	(3)	(2)	(5)	(6)	(1)
C Maximum pressure gradient (mmHg mm^{-1})		2.68	2.38	1.23	3.32	3.82 1.61
		(4)	(3)	(1)	(5)	(6) (2)

Values represent total ranks for all 20 subjects.
Values in parentheses indicate individual ranks for each parameter.
In all cases the χ^2 (df 5) statistic was significant at the 0.1 per cent level.

Table 17.3   Results of a Wilcoxon unplanned paired comparison of the differences between rank sum for any 2 support cushions

Parameter of pressure distribution	*Pairs of support cushions* 5–6	5–3	5–2	4–6	4–3	1–3	1–6
A Mean mmHg							
Difference	57	52.5	31.5	42	37.5	46.5	51
(df 6, 20)	**	**	n.s.	**	*	**	**
B Maximum mmHg							
Difference	77.5	73.5	45	54.5	50.5	46.5	50.5
(df 6, 20)	**	**	**	**	**	**	**
C Maximum pressure gradient (mmHg mm^{-1})							
Difference	62	72.5	40.5	48	58.5	40.5	30
(df 6, 20)	**	**	**	**	**	**	n.s.

n.s.: not significant; $*P<0.05$; $**P<0.01$.
The differences between rank sums were not significant for any of the other pairs of cushions.

cushions 5 and 3 and cushions 5 and 6 at the 1 per cent significance level.

On all support surfaces, each of the pressure parameters measured under the ischium was generally higher for the male group of subjects. However, when these parameters were corrected for body weight the differences were not significant at the 5 per cent level.

An inspection of the calculated parameters obtained on the plywood (support surface 7) revealed large variations both within individual subjects and between subjects. For example, the coefficient of variation between subjects ranged from 42 per cent to 55 per cent for the three pressure parameters. In 5 of the male subjects and 3 of the female subjects values of maximum pressure exceeding 300 mmHg (39.9 kPa) were obtained.

The results of the mechanical tests are illustrated in load versus

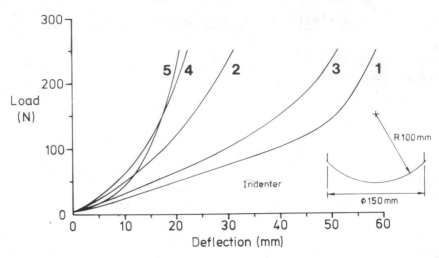

Figure 17.3 Load deformation behaviour under a spherical indenter of five support cushions

Table 17.4 Results of a Friedman analysis for each pair of cushions for all 10 subjects

Parameters of pressure distribution	Cushion cover materials				
	1–2	Terry 3–4	5–6	7–8	9–10
A Mean mmHg	27	32	30	28	33
	(1)	(4)	(3)	(2)	(5)
B Maximum mmHg	25	27	35	35.5	27.5
	(1)	(2)	(4)	(5)	(3)
C Maximum pressure gradient (mmHg mm^{-1})	28 (2)	31 (3)	32 (4)	36 (5)	23 (1)

Values represent total ranks for all 10 subjects.
Values in parentheses indicate individual ranks for each parameter.
In all cases the χ^2(df 4) statistic was not significant at the 5 per cent level.
Cushion arrangements 1, 3, 5, 7 and 9 include foam of support cushion 2, even cushion arrangements include foam of support cushion 3 (see Table 17.1).

deformation form in Figure 17.3. This reveals a considerable range of mechanical behaviour for the 5 tested cushions, although all exhibit a decrease in compliance at high levels of force.

Results of the analysis for the covered cushions indicated that there was no significant interaction at the 5 per cent level between covering materials and foam bases (Table 17.4).

DISCUSSION

Factors which affect the pressure distribution under the ischium when sitting include: subject weight and body build (Garber and Krouskop, 1982), the geometry of soft and bony tissues, the composition of the soft tissue and the mechanical properties of the various soft-tissue components (Bader and Bowker, 1983), and the geometry and mechanical properties of the support cushion. Analysis is complicated by the fact that further variation is introduced by postural changes, and variations in the mechanical properties of tissue and support surfaces with time.

In the present chapter, it has been possible to determine the relative importance of some of these variables with the aid of accurate measurements of pressure at the seating interface.

Support cushions with different mechanical properties would be expected to produce variations in pressure distribution under the ischium. However, an earlier study (Garber and Krouskop, 1982) found few clear and consistent differences between support surfaces, because the subjects varied widely in their responses. In the present study, a more controlled population of healthy normal subjects was investigated, and some consistent differences between support cushions were found, which could be related to the results of the mechanical tests. Cushions 3 and 5 showed large differences in the various parameters calculated from the pressure distribution, which could be attributed to their different mechanical stiffness, as illustrated by the load deflection curves (Figure 17.3). Overall, the results for cushion 5 were inconsistent with the expected behaviour of a gel cushion, which is intended to reduce high pressures by the redistribution of loads. Cushion 1 behaved in an anomalous fashion, exhibiting a low stiffness and yet producing high values of the pressure parameters. Careful examination showed, however, that at a typical mean pressure of 100 mmHg (13.3 kPa) the deformation of the cushion was 61 mm (80 per cent), a level sufficient to produce bottoming of the internal structure, indicated by the increasing slope of the load deflection curves. This must be considered when choosing both the stiffness and thickness of an appropriate support cushion.

Although the pressure parameters were found to differ significantly for some pairs of cushions, smaller differences between other pairs of cushions may none the less be of considerable clinical importance. It is well accepted that the process of tissue breakdown depends upon both the magnitude of applied pressure and its duration (Reswick and Rogers, 1976). Therefore even small differences in pressure distribution between cushions may be potentially damaging to the tissues in the long term. Further investigation is required before any guidelines can be produced to aid the selection of the most appropriate cushion for the individual patient.

Previous observations suggested that males are more prone to tissue breakdown than females (Cull and Smith, 1973). In the present study values of the three pressure parameters were significantly larger in male subjects, but when these parameters were corrected for body weight, the differences were not significant. Thus the increased values for male subjects could be attributed to a combination of body weight and sex, with the relative importance of each factor unknown.

The variable nature of the pressure distribution obtained with a subject sitting on the plywood surface probably reflected the relative movement of the soft-tissue layer adjacent to the ischial tuberosity. This finding demonstrates the difficulties of obtaining accurate and repeatable measurements of pressure distribution at a rigid support interface.

Accumulated results for all subjects revealed some significant differences in the pressure parameters obtained with the support surfaces. These findings confirmed that support surfaces with different mechanical properties produced variations in pressure distribution under the ischium. Continuation of the work may lead eventually to the establishment of guidelines for the choice of appropriate cushions for the individual patient in the seating clinic. There was often a preferential order of cushions for an individual subject. The individual order may be of clinical importance where one cushion is most suitable in terms of load distribution properties for an individual patient. In cases with very similar pressure-relieving properties, the choice of cushion would be determined by other functional and personal preference factors.

The results of the analysis for covered cushions suggest that the commonly available covers when used with different foams do not have a major effect on the pressure distribution under the ischium. However, it should be stressed that wrinkled or rucked materials at the seating interface would undoubtedly produce local increases in pressure distribution and should be always avoided.

The reported study has provided base line information on seating pressure distribution in a limited range of normal subjects. It may also be of some clinical use for comparison with test results from an age-matched group of spinal-injury patients. Other factors need to be investigated, including the effects of ageing on pressure distribution and the relationship between the pressure distribution and tissue blood flow (see Chapter 15) or other factors indicative of potential tissue breakdown.

ACKNOWLEDGEMENTS

We would like to thank Jon Gwillim, who designed and constructed the prototype Oxford Pressure Monitor, Carol Gant and Steve Riley for their help in carrying out the tests, Talley Medical Equipment who manufactured the sensor cell array, and all our volunteer subjects.

REFERENCES

Bader, D. L. and Bowker, P. (1983). Mechanical characteristics of skin and underlying tissues in vivo. *Biomaterials*, **4**, 305–308

Bader, D. L. and Hawken, M. B. (1986). Pressure distribution under the ischium of normal subjects. *J. Biomed. Eng.*, **8**, 353–357

Bader, D. L., Gwillim, J., Newson, T. P. and Harris, J. D. (1985). Pressure measurement at the patient support interface. In Whittle, M. W. and Harris, J. D. (eds), *Biomechanical Measurement in Orthopaedic Practice*, Oxford University Press, Oxford, pp. 145–150

Chow, W. W. and Odell, E. I. (1974). Deformation and stresses in soft body tissues of a sitting person. *J. Biomech. Eng.*, **100**, 79–87

Cochrane, G. M. and Wishere, E. R. (1988). In *Wheelchairs*, Equipment for the Disabled, Oxford, pp. 28–29

Colquhoun, D. (1971). In *Lectures on Biostatistics*, Clarendon, Oxford, pp. 209–210

Cull, J. G. and Smith, O. H. (1973). A preliminary note on demographic and personality correlates on decubitus ulcer incidence. *J. Psychol.*, **85**, 225–227

Denne, W. A. (1981). The 'hammock' effect in wheelchair cushion covers. *Paraplegia*, **19**, 38–42

Engel, P. (1988). Pressure distribution on cushions in canvas wheelchairs and in wheelchairs with stable, contoured seat forms. In Bougie, T. and Davies, A. (eds), *Wheelchairs: Research, Evaluation and Development*, COMAC BME, Milan, pp. 125–134

Ferguson-Pell, M. W. (1980). Design criteria for the measurement at body/support interfaces. *Eng. Med.*, **9**, 209–214

Ferguson-Pell, M. W., Cochran, G. V. B., Palmieri, V. R. and Brunski, J. B. (1986). Development of a modular wheelchair cushion for spinal cord injury persons. *J. Rehab. Res. Dev.*, **23**, 63–76

Garber, S. L. and Krouskop, T. A. (1982). Body build and its relationship to pressure distribution in the seated wheelchair patient. *Arch. Phys. Med. Rehab.*, **63**, 17–20

Garber, S. L., Krouskop, T. A. and Carter, R. E. (1978). System for clinically evaluating wheelchair pressure-relief cushions. *Am. J. Occup. Ther.*, **32**, 565–570

Husain, T. (1953). An experimental study of some pressure effects on tissue with reference to the bed sore problem. *J. Path. Bact.*, **66**, 347–358

Jay, P. (1983). In *Choosing the Best Wheelchair Cushion*, Royal Association for Disability and Rehabilitation, London, pp. 1–8

Krouskop, T. A., Williams, R., Noble, P. and Brown, J. (1986). Inflation pressure effect on performance of air-filled wheelchair cushions. *Arch. Phys. Med. Rehabil.*, **67**, 126–128

Landis, E. M. (1930). Micro-injection studies of capillary blood pressure in human skin. *Heart*, **15**, 209–228

Reddy, N. P., Cochran, G. V. B. and Krouskop, T. A. (1981). Interstitial fluid flow as a factor in decubitus ulcer formation. *J. Biomechanics*, **14**, 879–81

Reswick, J. B. and Rogers, J. E. (1976). Experiences at Los Amigos Hospital with devices and techniques to prevent pressure sores. In Kenedi, R. M., Cowden, J. M. and Scales, J. T. (eds), *Bed Sore Biomechanics*, Macmillan Press, London and Basingstoke, pp. 301–310

Riley, S. and Bader, D. L. (1988). Biomechanical measurements of back shape and interface pressures in unsupported sitting. *Clin. Biomechanics*, **3**, 114–117

Scales, J. (1982). Pressure sore prevention. *Care, Science and Practice*, **1**, 9–17

18

Pressure Management and the Recumbent Person

Thomas A. Krouskop, Susan L. Garber and Philip Noble

INTRODUCTION

As the mobility of a growing segment of our society becomes impaired through either trauma or advancing age, soft-tissue breakdown, or pressure sores, become an increasingly provocative problem. Preventing pressure sores in the elderly or in victims of trauma who suffer from reduced mobility requires a programme that successfully co-ordinates technological and medical expertise. Knowledge of pressure sore etiology provides a framework for designing a programme that adapts technology to the individual's lifestyle.

LIMITATIONS OF BIOMECHANICAL STUDIES OF TISSUE BREAKDOWN

The scientific studies that have advanced our knowledge of the factors involved in the formation of pressure sores have also provided a basis for improving preventive techniques. Most of these studies have focused on the biomechanical aspects of pressure sore formation. A number of investigators have studied blood flow and tissue mechanics in attempts to quantify the relationship between externally applied loads and the internal stresses that stop blood flow. In Kosiak's classic study (1959) the variables governing soft-tissue breakdown were extended to include 'time at pressure'. While Kosiak's relationship between 'time at pressure' and breakdown is associated with considerable variance, Rogers (1973) proved its clinical significance. As these early studies became well publicised, investigators began to appreciate that tissue breakdown was probably a multidimensional process. The variables identified included pressure, shear loading, general metabolic condition of the person, local tissue integrity and viability, age, oedema, repeated pressure, altered sensation, neurotrophic effects, and psychosocial factors (Williams, 1972). Unfortunately, most studies have isolated only one or two of the variables for examination, leaving the other variables uncontrolled or assumed to be constant, even though other investigators have identified them as significant contributing factors. For example, the age, metabolic condition and levels of general neuroendocrine stress in subjects (human and animal) have not been controlled in most studies.

EXTERNALLY APPLIED PRESSURE

Although control of the shearing load applied is a critical variable, the shape of the load applicators has been studied only recently (Brunski, 1984). Many of these studies have been designed with animal models. Typically, the animals have been subjected to various externally applied pressure loads using indenters of different geometric forms. As a result, substantial data have been collected indicating that pressures of at least 200 mmHg (26 kPa) are necessary to produce tissue breakdown (Cochran, 1980; Dinsdale, 1973; Ryan, 1979; Seiler and Stahelin, 1979). Consequently, it is difficult, often impossible, to compare directly the results obtained in one laboratory with those from another. General trends may be noted, but valuable specific values are often found to be incompatible.

Several studies have been conducted to elucidate the relationship between externally applied pressure and cessation of blood flow in a region, some by analysing soft-tissue oxygenation (Grounds, 1973; Artigue and Hyman, 1976). Studies based on the most widely used model, the Krough cylinder, have produced useful information for determining where, when, and for how long blood flow will cease after an area has been loaded with externally applied pressure. The animal studies indicate that 'healthy' tissue can withstand pressure of 300 mmHg (40 kPa) (Cochran, 1980) for periods up to 18 hours with reversible damage. Unfortunately, the magnitude of the pressure and load duration time typically derived from those studies are inconsistent with conditions existing in a hospital or nursing-home setting. Consequently, investigators have started to look for additional factors causing blood cessation and/or tissue damage.

SHEAR STRESS

Bennett *et al.* (1979) and Reichel (1958) have researched the role of shear stress in pressure sore formation. Their work indicates that shear forces can add significantly to the effect of externally applied normal forces in occluding blood flow in soft tissue. Bennett theorised that in addition to friction, large gradients in normal stresses produce shear forces that severely damage soft tissues. He concluded that although shear force plays a significant part in the occlusion of blood vessels, shear stress alone cannot break down tissue; a sufficiently occlusive shear condition develops only under large compressive forces. His work indicates however that the pressure level capable of disrupting blood flow can be reduced by one-half with the presence of significant shear forces.

REPETITIVE STRESS

Brand (1976) has contributed most to our knowledge about the effects of repetitive stress on soft tissue. Rats have been used as the model animals to study the effects of low-magnitude pressure as a cause of soft-tissue breakdown in several studies (Manley and Darby, 1980). In Brand's experiments, repetitive subcritical loads were applied to the rat's foot pad in different patterns over a period of 3 weeks. These loadings created necrotic areas in the soft tissue that had characteristics similar to those of pressure sores. Of particular importance was the finding that during the stressing of soft tissue, the introduction of rest intervals followed by restressing caused the soft-tissue regions to hypertrophy and become capable of bearing much greater external loads than before. On the basis of Brand's work, design criteria have been developed and used in the fabrication of shoes for persons with insensitive or severely deformed feet as found in Hansen's disease, peripheral neuropathies, and the peripheral vascular disorders associated with diabetes.

METABOLIC CONDITION

Krouskop and Garber (1981) hypothesised that the accumulation of waste products, as well as deficits in metabolic nutrient supply in a region of tissue, may be primary factors in producing pressure sores. Analytical and experimental studies have been conducted to investigate the effects of altered lymphatic drainage on the formation of pressure sores. These are detailed in Chapter 16.

Several investigators have noted the influence of psychosocial factors on the incidence of decubitus ulcers. The individual's responsibility for his or her own skin care and satisfaction with the activities of life have some correlation with the risk of skin ulceration (Manley, 1978; Moolton, 1973). Understanding of the causes and risks of skin breakdown, combined with a positive attitude towards health and independent living, are also expected to influence heavily the effects of potentially dangerous mechanical factors in everyday life.

GENERAL MEDICAL CONDITION

Susceptibility to pressure sores is also related to the general medical condition of the individual (Manley, 1978). Incontinence, for example, has long been associated with decubitus ulcers. In the Greater Glasgow Health Board Survey, while 3.7 per cent of continent patients had significant pressure sores, the incidence rose to 15.5 per cent and 39.7 per cent among those with urinary and faecal incontinence respectively (Jordan and Clark, 1977). The observation must be attributed, in part, to the susceptibility of moist skin to maceration through direct trauma or exposure to pressure. Also, wet skin is more likely to adhere to clothing and bed linens, thus enhancing the generation of substantial shearing forces. An additional factor in faecal incontinence is the mechanical attribution of the epidermis combined with the introduction of infection into any breach of the body's defences.

Poor nutrition, resulting in loss of weight and reduced padding of the bony prominences, is another important factor (Williams, 1972). The body's normal tissue integrity is dependent upon a correct nitrogen balance and vitamin intake. Hypoproteinaemia leading to oedema causes the skin to become less elastic and more susceptible to inflammation as the rate of oxygen transfer from the capillaries to the tissue is reduced, thus compromising the skin's viability.

Recently, the role of skin temperature and perspiration in the process of soft tissue breakdown has become an active area of pressure sore research (Mahanty and Roemer, 1979; Van der Leun *et al.*, 1974).

The soft tissue may be modelled as an enzyme-activated chemical engine wherein slight changes in the operating temperature environment, particularly temperature increases, produce dramatic effects by increasing the metabolic demands of the cells in the local region. A rise of 2 °C can change the metabolic demands by as much as an order of magnitude.

Similarly, the use of hypothermia to reduce the metabolic demands of a region, and the use of temperature as a predictive tool, have been explored in several laboratories. In one study, infrared thermography has been employed to study thermal changes in the skin related to the effects of repetitive stresses and to monitor the healing rate of established sores (Cochran, 1980). Mahanty and Roemer (1979) have also contributed new knowledge on how temperature affects soft tissue breakdown.

Unfortunately, many of the research results have not been effectively translated into clinically useful formats. Furthermore, there are still many oversimplified and misleading notions about pressure sores that limit the effectiveness of preventive programmes. This results in the ineffective use of technological aids developed to help reduce the occurrence of pressure sores.

CONSIDERATIONS IN SELECTING SUPPORT SURFACES

An important component of a tissue pressure management programme is selecting support surfaces that reduce peak pressure and control the pressure gradients that exist in the soft tissue when a person sits or lies in a bed. Inadequate management too often results from the incorrect assumption that if tissue pressure is kept below 32 mmHg (4.3 kPa), the average value of capillary pressure for healthy adults reported in physiology texts, pressure sores will not form. This simplistic view is inconsistent with the results of previous studies. Although lack of blood flow to a region can cause tissue death, the experimental time required for such damage to occur seems to be much longer than the actual time associated with tissue breakdown in clinical environments. A primary factor in the breakdown of soft tissue is the flow of interstitial fluid out of the region and the subsequent microvascular damage that occurs. Interstitial fluid flow is controlled by pressure gradients across the tissue and the resistance to flow offered by the soft tissue matrix. Moreover, Bennett and co-workers (1979) have demonstrated that capillary pressures in the buttocks of seated geriatric subjects who have peripheral vascular disease may be as low as 8–12 mmHg (1.1–1.6 kPa). The physics of the support problem, i.e. the weight of a person's body divided by the projected area available to support the body, precludes the possibility of having all pressures less than 10 mmHg (1.3 kPa), even for a supine person.

In order to select the most effective support surface for an individual, it is important to recognise that no single threshold pressure can insure tissue viability for every individual (see Figure 15.2). Consequently, the best compromise is to select support surfaces that reduce interface pressures to a minimum. This selection process can be facilitated by ranking the effectiveness of products according to how well they reduce the pressures experienced on a hard, flat surface, how long they last, and how much they cost. Many companies have developed a plethora of new devices aimed at providing 'the ideal support medium'. Unfortunately, without an understanding of the aetiology of soft-tissue breakdown, the definition of an ideal support medium is impossible.

Pressure sore prevention programmes often expend considerable resources on providing patients with wheelchair cushions that redistribute body weight away from bony prominences during sitting (see Chapter 17). Often however there is little discussion about the bed surface that supports the patients when they are not in the wheelchair. Selecting a support surface that provides stability for the skeleton and controls the distribution of the body weight requires ingenuity and judicious use of materials such as foams or air mattresses. An adequate surface should distribute body weight over the maximum area to reduce the pressures in the tissues and should control the shear forces that are generated on the skin surface.

Ideally, during recumbency the pressures on the soft tissue should be reduced to 30 mmHg (4 kPa) or less, since the hydrostatic pressure generated in this posture does not significantly contribute to the forces that tend to maintain flow of blood and lymph. When a person is recumbent, variability in the body surface contours is more exaggerated than when the person is seated, leading to the need for a support surface that is capable of large deformations without generating large restoring forces.

The deformation requirements for a bed support surface are dictated by the differences in elevations between the lumbar areas of the back and the coccygeal region when the person is supine, and the differences between the waist and trochanters when the person is lying on his side. If the support surface is not able to accommodate deformation of a magnitude permitting prominent areas to sink into the support, the area available for weight-bearing is reduced in the region and the pressures tending to impede the transport phenomena are increased.

Mattresses and Beds

There are four basic groups of static mattress overlays: foam, gel, water-filled and air-filled systems. Each type of system has inherent advantages and disadvantages, which are summarized in Table 18.1.

When the user has significant complications or is at high risk of developing pressure problems, or quality nursing care cannot be assured, it may be advantageous to consider one of the air flotation bed systems. There are two types that are popular, the low-air-loss bed and the air-fluidised bed. Depending on the needs of the individual who is placed on the bed and the availability of service personnel to maintain the equipment, one type will generally be more suitable than the other.

The advantages of the air-fluidised bed include ease of operation, relative immunity to power failure, and control of skin maceration. Its primary limitations are heavy weight and limited positioning and posturing of the patient without the use of cushions.

Because the low-air-loss beds are comfortable, control skin maceration and enable easy change in posture, these products require personnel who can adjust the air flow in order to make them effective tools for pressure sore prevention. Another disadvantage is the need for back-up power; the air bags deflate if the power fails and no longer provide protection.

It should be noted that in testing in the rehabilitation engineering programme at The Texax Institute for Rehabilitation and Research (TIRR), the interface pressure readings on all of the air-fluidised beds and low-air-loss beds were found to provide interface pressures that were not statistically different from each other, as long as care was taken to adjust the low-air-loss products. Without proper adjustment these products

Table 18.1 Characteristics of support systems

Type	Advantages	Disadvantages
Air-filled	1. Lightweight 2. Cleanable	1. Subject to puncture 2. Not easily repairable 3. Air pressure must be checked against leakage and for proper regulation
Water-filled	1. Cleanable 2. Relatively inexpensive	1. Heavy 2. Subject to puncture
Flotation gel	1. Adjusts to body's movement 2. Simulates body fat tissue to provide more padding between patient and bed surface	1. Heavy 2. Difficult to transfer 3. Must be stored flat
Polymer foams	1. Very readily available 2. Large variety of types 3. Inexpensive 4. Lightweight 5. Easily transferred 6. Can be cut into any size, shape, thickness 7. Can be modified	1. Wear out more quickly than other materials 2. Not cleanable 3. Effected by changes in climate and temperature 4. Should not be used or stored in direct sunlight

provided less protection than the static systems.

In another study at TIRR, 9 commercially available mattress overlay systems and 30 geriatric foam overlays were evaluated. A standard hospital mattress with a Staph-check cover was used during each testing session as a control surface and as the foundation for all the overlays. The generic foam overlays of different densities and thicknesses were produced from polyurethane foam that had a 25 per cent indentation load deflection (ILD) of 32 lbf (142.3 N). Half of the samples were solid foam overlays and the other half were convoluted samples. The commercial products were provided by the manufacturers and were set for operation according to the instructions sent by the suppliers. The commercially available products included the following:

1. Stryker mattress overlay – foam overlay with gel-filled inserts
2. 50 mm thick convoluted foam overlay
3. 100 mm thick convoluted foam overlay
4. Gaymar Sof-Care overlay – an air-filled system
5. Roho overlay – a segmented air-filled product
6. Akros mattress – a combination of foam and gel that replaces the conventional mattress

7. Span America Geomatt overlay – an 89 mm thick foam overlay that is constructed to provide different stiffness (ILD) for the head, torso and legs
8. Gaymar alternating air pad – a tubular air-filled overlay that alternately inflates and deflates adjacent tubes
9. Lapidus alternating air pad – a tubular air-filled overlay that has a 25 mm foam cover. The air tubes alternately inflate and deflate.

Thirty subjects selected from the population available at TIRR and the Spinal Cord Unit at the Veterans Administration Medical Center in Houston were tested on the commercially available products. Another sample of 32 subjects from TIRR were tested on the generic foam overlays. The subjects were categorized by sex and by body build defined in terms of age, height and weight. Each of the subjects was tested while lying on his or her back and side so that interface pressures could be monitored under the scapulae, the sacral-coccygeal area, and the trochanteric area.

Subjects wearing loose-fitting clothing were told to remove all objects from their pockets and to remove their belts and shoes before being evaluated. Subjects wearing tight clothes with double seams were instructed to change into a surgical scrub suit before the testing session.

A transducer pad was placed between the mattress and the area of the subject's body to be monitored. Bony prominences were palpated, and the locations were noted on the data collection form. Maximum pressure for each of the prominences was then recorded. To improve the reproducibility and the accuracy of the peak pressure measurements, the readings were taken 3 times and the average of the 3 readings was recorded for each bony prominence.

Position while lying on the side was standardised for all subjects using a goniometer to position the hips in 45° of flexion. The trunk was positioned perpendicular to the support surface. Each subject was instructed not to move while the readings were being taken. During scapular and sacral pressure measurements the subjects' arms were placed flat along their sides.

Results of the study were based on an analysis of the maximum pressure measured under the bony prominences on all the support surfaces.

Figures 18.1 to 18.3 show the mean peak pressures under the trochanter, sacrum and scapulae for each of the commercially available mattress overlays. For the Lapidus and Gaymar models, both the high and low readings in the cycle are represented on the graphs.

An analysis of the statistical significance of the differences between the standard mattress (control) and the therapeutic mattress overlays was conducted using Student's t-test. When compared with the standard mattress, all the therapeutic mattresses provided a reduction and redistribution of pressure under the trochanter and the sacrum ($p < 0.01$).

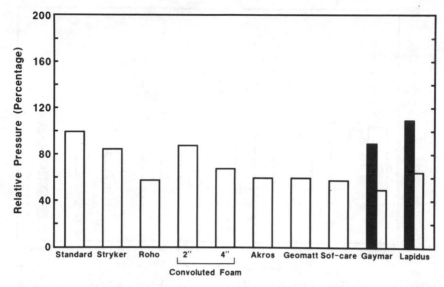

Figure 18.1 Interface pressures under the trochanter. Values are normalised to the mean peak pressure measured on the standard mattress

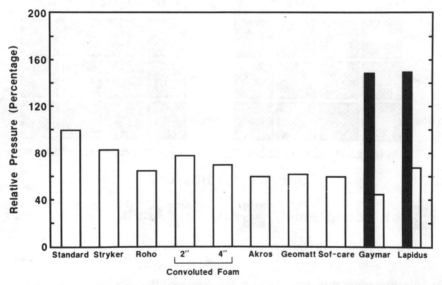

Figure 18.2 Interface pressures under the sacral–coccygeal area. Values are normalised to the mean peak pressures measured on the standard mattress

On all mattresses, maximum pressures under the trochanter and sacrum were generally lower for women than for men. There was no difference in scapular pressure readings between men and women. Very similar pressure curves were seen for thin, average-weight and heavy subjects, with all the

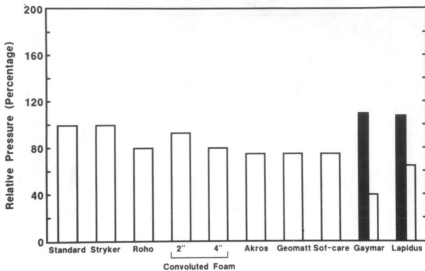

Figure 18.3 Interface pressures under the scapula. Values are normalised to the mean peak pressures measured on the standard mattress

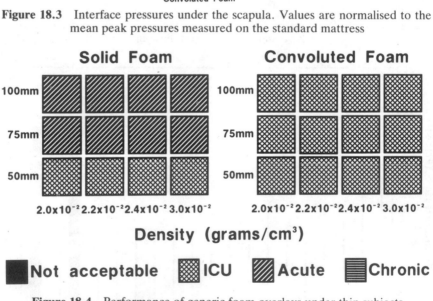

Figure 18.4 Performance of generic foam overlays under thin subjects

trends remaining the same. In fact, the relative effectiveness of each of the overlays was independent of the body build of the user.

Figures 18.4 to 18.6 summarise the results of the testing done on the generic foam overlays. The convoluted samples were typical of many commercial products. The 50-mm samples had 1.3-mm bases; the 75-mm had 1.9-mm bases; and the 100-mm had 1.9-mm bases. Using the criteria given in Table 18.2, the overlays were rated for their potential use in

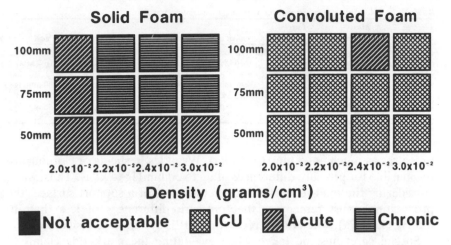

Figure 18.5 Performance of generic foam overlays under average subjects

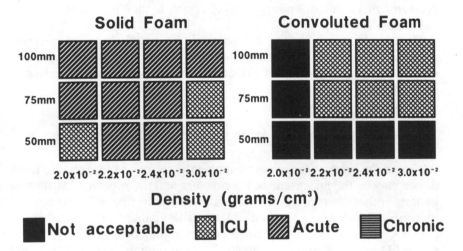

Figure 18.6 Performance of generic foam overlays under heavy subjects

various environments. These criteria are based on the allowable time at a given pressure under each of the bony areas monitored during the data-collection process. The allowable pressures were determined from the Reswick and Rogers pressure curve and the clinical experience of the TIRR rehabilitation engineering department.

The allowable pressures vary according to environment in which the mattress overlay is used; see Table 18.2.

Experience at TIRR also indicates that even minor muscle contractions and changes in posture can lead to variations in interface pressure of 8–12 mmHg (1.1–1.6 kPa). Spasticity in muscles can change peak interface

Table 18.2   Allowable interface pressures according to use environment

Use environment	Max. use length	Care frequency	Scapula	Sacroccygeal	Trochanter	Heel
ICU	7 days	Hourly, with side positioning	45 mmHg (6 kPa)	45 mmHg (6 kPa)	70 mmHg (9.3 kPa)	50 mmHg (6.7 kPa)
acute care	21 days	2 hour	40 mmHg (5.3 kPa)	40 mmHg (5.3 kPa)	50 mmHg (6.7 kPa)	50 mmHg (6.7 kPa)
chronic care	6 months	6–8 hour	35 mmHg (4.7 kPa)	35 mmHg (4.7 kPa)	45 mmHg (6 kPa)	45 mmHg (6 kPa)

pressures as much as 45 mmHg (6 kPa). Wrinkles in sheets or clothing are responsible for pressure differences of up to 30 mmHg (4 kPa). Thus, when considering the load-redistributing effectiveness of a support surface, the professional must remember that pressure differences of less than 10 mmHg (1.3 kPa), when measured with a TIPE system, are insignificant.

Special care must be taken when evaluating the marketing claims of manufacturers of products designed to reduce differences in average pressures of less than 9 mmHg (1.2 kPa) unless they represent averages based on a very large sample.

Therefore, when selecting a support surface, differences in interface pressures of less than 10 mmHg (1.3 kPa) should be considered to provide equally effective pressure redistribution for care purposes, and selection should be based on other factors.

PATIENT DIAGNOSIS AND LIFESTYLE CONSIDERATIONS

Although the primary factors determining the selection of a pressure relief device may be the magnitude of the pressure and the pressure distribution pattern, other factors contribute significantly to the effectiveness of pressure relief devices. The first of these is the patient's diagnosis. Is the person's disability secondary to disease, trauma, or immobility due to ageing? Does the person have intact, absent or diminished sensation in the anatomical areas vulnerable to breakdown? The number of hours spent on the support surfaces and the scheduling pattern of those hours are also important considerations when deciding on a device. Does the person sit for one long, extended period or does he sit for shorter periods with rests in between each sitting period? What types of activities does he perform? These may include self-care, vocational, educational, homemaking, re-creational and social activities. Each activity will vary the patient's position and each will exert different levels of pressure and stress on the soft tissues.

Another factor that should be considered when selecting a pressure relief system for a person with a physical disability is the usage environment of the equipment. The climate, levels of pollution and humidity, and the patient's continence, will have an effect on some of the materials of which pressure relief devices are made. For example, some of the foams are affected by severe changes in temperature. These devices also retain odours and cannot be washed or adequately cleaned.

The self-sufficiency of a person's living arrangement is another important consideration in selection. Is the person living alone and totally independent or is he assisted by family members, friends, attendants, or nurses? If the support system is very heavy or requires frequent maintenance, it would be inappropriate for the person who does not have access to assistance.

Long- and short-term tissue histories are excellent indicators of the effectiveness of pressure-relief devices. Has the person ever had pressure sores or surgery to correct a pressure sore?

Moreover, body build has been shown to influence pressure distribution in the person seated in a wheelchair (Garber and Krouskop, 1982). Thinner persons have higher pressures under bony prominences more frequently than do individuals of average or heavier weights. For this reason, thinner persons may bottom out on the softer cushions.

It must be recognised that optimal application of technological advances requires the exercising of considerable judgement. Technology is an alternative form of assistance that can provide disabled people with quality care while reducing the need for attendant care.

REFERENCES

Artigue, R. S. and Hyman, W. A. (1976). The effect of myoglobin on the oxygen concentration in skeletal muscle subjected to ischaemia. *Annl. Biomed. Eng.*, **4**(2), 128–137

Bennett, L., Kauver, D., Lee, B. Y. and Trainor, F. A. (1979). Shear vs pressure as causative factors in skin blood flow occlusion. *Arch. Phys. Med. Rehabil.*, **60**, 309–314

Brand, P. W. (1976). Pressure sores. In Kenedi, R. M., Cowden, J. M. and Scales, J. T. (eds), *Bed Sore Biomechanics*, Macmillan Press, London and Basingstoke, pp. 19–25

Brunski, J. B. (1984). Pressure sores: biomechanics of indented tissues. *Proc. 37th ACEMB, Los Angeles, CA, Sept. 1984*, p. 181

Cochran, G. V. B. (1980). The pig as a model for soft tissue experiments. Presented at the Workshop on the Effects of Mechanical Stress on Soft Tissues, Dallas, Texas, Nov. 5–7, 1980. (No published record.)

Dinsdale, S. M. (1973). Decubitus ulcers in swine: light and electron microscopy study of pathogenesis. *Arch. Phys. Med. Rehabil.*, **45**, 51–56

Garber, S. L. and Krouskop, T. A. (1982). Body build and its relationship to pressure distribution in the seated wheelchair patient. *Arch. Phys. Med. Rehabil.*, **63**, 17–20

Grounds, D. (1973). A Model to Predict Oxygen Tension in a Capillary-Tissue System Subjected to Periodic Occlusion. Masters Thesis, Texas A & M University

Jordan, M. M. and Clark, M. (1977). Report on Incidance of Pressure Sores in the Patient Community of the Greater Glasgow Health Board Area, University of Strathclyde, January 21

Kosiak M. (1959). Etiology and pathology of ischemic ulcers. *Arch. Phys. Med. Rehabil.*, **40**, 62–69

Krouskop, T. A. and Garber, S. L. (1981). A Synthesis of the Factors that Contribute to Pressure Sore Formation. Presented at NATO Advanced Study Institute in Spinal Cord Injury Rehabilitation Engineering, Stoke Mandeville Hospital, Aylesbury, England, May 11–23

Krouskop, T. A., Noble, P. C., Garber, S. L. and Spencer, W. A. (1983). The effectiveness of preventive management in reducing the occurrence of pressure sores. *J. of Rehab. R & D*, **20**, 74–83

Mahanty, S. D. and Roemer, R. B. (1979). Thermal response of skin to application of localized pressure. *Arch. Phys. Med. Rehabil.*, **60**, 584–590

Manley, M. T. (1978). Incidence, contributory factors, and costs of pressure sores. *South African Med. J.*, **53**(6), 217–222

Manley, M. T. and Darby, T. (1980). Repetitive mechanical stress and denervation in plantar ulcer pathogenesis in rats. *Arch. Phys. Med. Rehabil.*, **61**, 171–177

Moolton, S. E. (1973). Suggestions on the prevention and management of bed sores. *Med. Times.*, **101**(6), 52–56

Reddy, N. P. and Cochran, G. V. B. (1979). Phenomenological theory underlying pressure–time relationship in decubitus ulcer formation. *Federation Proc.*, **38** (2), 1153

Reichel, S. M. (1958). Shear force as a factor in decubitus ulcers in paraplegics, *J. Am. Med. Assoc.*, **166**, 762–763

Rogers, J. E. (1973). *Annual Report of the Rehabilitation Engineering Center*, Rancho Los Amigos Hospital, Downey, California

Ryan, T. J. (1979). Blood supply and decubitus ulcers. *Int. J. Dermatology*, **18**, 123–124

Seiler, W. P. and Stahelin, H. B. (1979). Skin oxygen tension as a function of imposed skin pressure–implication for decubitus ulcer formation. *J. Amer. Geriatric Soc.*, **27**(7), 298–301

Van Der Leun, J. E., Lowe, L. B., Jr and Beerens E. G. J. (1974). The influence of skin temperature on dermal–epidermal adherence: evidence compatible with a highly viscous bond. *J. Investigative Dermatol*, **16**(1), 42–46

Williams, A. (1972). A study of factors contributing to skin breakdown, *Nursing Reg.*, **21**(3), 238–243

19

Movement Studies During Sleep

J. C. Barbenel

INTRODUCTION

The development of a pressure sore has important implications for the person with the sore, and for the medical and nursing care which the patient will require. A major priority in the care of patients at risk of developing sores must be prevention. The process leading to the development of a sore is complex, but the initiation is usually related to tissue trauma produced by mechanical forces acting on the skin and the subcutaneous tissue.

Animal experiments in which tissue trauma has been produced by the application of pressure show that both the magnitude of the applied force and the time for which it is applied are important (Daniel *et al.*, 1981, which contains additional references). In general, the greater the pressure the shorter the time for which it need be applied to produce tissue damage. Data on human pressure sores are necessarily more limited, but retrospective investigations of patients who have developed pressure sores confirm, in a general way, the results of animal experiments and the importance of the interaction of pressure magnitude and duration in sore production (Reswick and Rogers, 1976).

People with normal sensation and mobility avoid tissue trauma by frequent movements, which reposition the body segments and redistribute the forces acting on the tissues. Restricted mobility has been shown epidemiologically to be associated with a high prevalence of pressure sores, examples being para- or tetraplegic patients (Noble, 1981) and the elderly (Barbenel *et al.*, 1977; Jordan and Barbenel, 1983). The replacement of spontaneous body movements in bed by regular manual turning or by active support systems such as ripple mattresses, are well-established and effective methods of pressure sore prevention, but are costly in manpower or finance, and cannot be made available to all patients. Consequently the detection of patients at high risk of developing pressure sores and the preferential allocation of scarce resources to these patients are important components of any regimen for the prevention of pressure sores.

The recognition of the relationship between pressure sore risk and the ability or extent of movement has led to the incorporation of mobility in clinical scoring systems for pressure sore risk assessment. In the well-known Norton scoring system (Norton *et al.*, 1962) there are two factors which describe the movement potential of the patient. Mobility is classified as full, slightly limited, very limited or immobile and the associated factor of activity is classified as ambulant, walks with help, chairbound or bedbound. The distinctions in the activity classification are clear, but the subdivisions of the mobility classification are rather more subjective. Alternative risk assessment systems (e.g. Lowthian, 1987) have modified the nature of the question relating to mobility but still require a subjective assessment by the scorer.

TECHNIQUES FOR THE MEASUREMENT OF MOVEMENTS IN BED

Methods and systems for the measurement of the movement of subjects in bed were initially developed to investigate sleep and the physiological and psychological factors which influence it. Many of these devices were non-electrical, depending in some cases on ingenious arrangements of strings and pulleys and utilising tambours as recording devices. The early systems are reviewed by Kleitman (1932). They are almost entirely of historical interest, but they represent the precursor of systems and principles of measurement which have been subsequently refined or reinvented, in a more convenient format.

There are three general techniques which have been used to measure movement in bed: detection of the movement of the body or body segments by transducers attached to the subject, the monitoring of some aspect of the bed which can be related to the subject position, direct observation or recording of the total posture of the subject.

Transducers Attached to the Subject

Trunk movement has been monitored by attaching transducers to the subject's sternum. Kresse and Rettenmaier (1973) described a weighted rotary potentiometer transducer, and Korn *et al.* (1974) a weighted accelerometer. Smaller versions of these two devices have been developed for attachment to the extremities, usually being worn round the wrist or ankle.

A similar device specifically designed to investigate mobility in relation to pressure sores was described by Bar *et al.* (1983). The sensor consisted of two mercury tilt switches at 120° to each other, which were encapsulated in rubber. The completed assembly was fixed to the mid-line of the trunk of the experimental subject. Initial results were reported for both spinal-cord-injured patients and normal subjects.

Movement records are also obtained as a by-product during the monitoring of interface pressures and temperature. Barbenel *et al.* (1978) used three arrays of thin, flexible pressure sensors (Ferguson-Pell *et al.*, 1976), which incorporated thermistors. The sensors were located over the right and left trochanters and the sacrum, and scanned at 10-minute intervals during the subject's sleep. The results (Figure 19.1) showed that the pressure history indicated periods of load relief and intensification, related to the subject's movement. The temperature trace was consistent with the pressure history but was far less useful in detecting movements because of the presence of elevated temperatures after the tissues beneath the thermistor had been unloaded, probably produced by reactive hyperaemia (see Chapter 12). The monitoring was carried out on several consecutive nights (Wheatley, 1982), and the results very strongly suggest that the presence of the sensors and associated leads modify the movement patterns of the subject. The perturbing effect is likely to occur in all subject-mounted sensors, and is a very undesirable feature militating against the use of such devices.

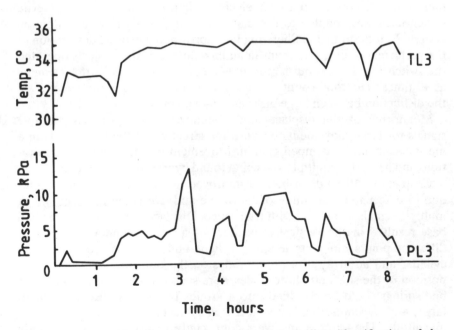

Figure 19.1   Measurements of trochanteric pressure allow identification of the time at which movements are made. The temperature records are consistent with the pressure but less useful for detecting movements. Data obtained from normal subjects

Monitoring the Bed

The movements of patients in bed can be monitored by detecting the effect of the subject movement on the bed itself. The use of an array of temperature sensors to identify the position of the patient on the bed surface has been suggested (Tamura *et al.*, 1988), but mechanical effects have been used more commonly.

Displacement

Most techniques using the bed to monitor patient movement rely on the deformation of the support surface. Many of the devices utilise the displacement of the mesh bed base supporting the mattress.

Cox and Marley (1959) described a device in which vertical displacements of the bed base in the region of the hips and shoulders actuated a potentiometer which produced electrical signals suitable for subsequent conditioning, analysis and recording. A simpler system, specifically designed to investigate the interrelationship between mobility and pressure sores, was described by Sherwin *et al.* (1961). The system was based on an inertia switch connected to an electrical impulse counter. The inertia switch itself was coupled to the mattress springing via a rack-and-pinion system. Exton-Smith and Sherwin (1961) provided a general description of the performance of the system. Small movements of the subjects operated the switch 1 or 2 times but larger movements actuated the switch as many as 12 times. The total count was used as a mobility index, irrespective of the distinction between large and small movements.

Monitoring of the displacement of mattress base provides multiple signals for large movements because the structure of the bed results in a mechanically under-damped system. Movement produces sustained vibrations and hence the multiple switching found by Exton-Smith and Sherwin.

Crisp *et al.* (1970) described an improved displacement-sensing technique to detect the magnitude of the move and overcome the problem of multiple signals associated with transience. Displacement of the spring bed base resulted in the vertical movement of a brass cylinder with slits at different points along its length. A light bulb was located within the cylinder and an array of 4 photodiodes on the outside of the tube. The position of the slits and photodiodes were such that the depression of the bed springs could be classified into 4 groups from small displacement to large, and by implication interpreted as subject movements of different magnitude. The photodiodes were connected in pairs to ensure that only the equilibrium displacement was recorded and not the oscillatory transients. The authors validated the technique with normal subjects. It is clear from their results that the weight of the subjects strongly affected the bed spring displacement, and the output of the device had to be scaled or corrected for subject weight.

There is little doubt that the measurement of bed spring displacement provides a method for detecting both the number and magnitude of subject movements in bed. The current King's Fund bed base is, however, solid rather than a spring mesh and the displacements are very much smaller, making such devices unusable for the overwhelming majority of hospital beds in present use.

A displacement-measuring device incorporated into the upper surface of the mattress, and therefore independent of the type of bed base, has been described by Brocklehurst *et al.* (1974). Twelve straight, parallel, soft rubber tubes containing water from a reservoir were fitted in a sheet covering the mattress. The tubes were connected to the reservoir by a non-return valve, and each time a tube was compressed by subject movement the water it contained was displaced into a collecting vessel, the height of the water in the vessel being continuously monitored. The output was related to the magnitude of the movements made, but the overall output trace was characterised in terms of the sums of the squares of the inter-move intervals, irrespective of the move magnitude. The results indicate very clearly that during the first 3 nights of monitoring the mobility patterns changed, confirming the perturbing influence of the presence of the system, similar to that noted above for pressure sensors.

Force Transmitted by the Bed

The weight of a person in bed is carried by the four bed legs. The distribution of the forces between the legs depends on the position of the centre of mass of the person relative to the bed itself. Movements will alter this position and the changes in posture and position produced by movements can be identified by measuring the loads transmitted by the legs. This allows the occurrence of a movement to be both detected and quantified.

If a subject of weight W on a bed of width w and length l moves such that the position of their centre of mass is displaced by distance d then there will be a change ΔF_s in the sum of forces transmitted by legs on the same side of the bed, and also a change ΔF_f in the sum of the forces transmitted via the legs at the foot of the bed. The distance d is related to these variables by the following equation:

$$d = \frac{[(w\,\Delta F_s)^2 + (l\,\Delta F_f)^2]^{1/2}}{W}.$$

The technique has been implemented by Barbenel *et al.* (1986), who supported each of the legs of a King's Fund bed on specially developed, low-profile load cells (Wheatley *et al.*, 1982). The analogue output of each cell was digitised and logged using a microcomputer system.

The results once again showed that beds are less than ideal transducer systems. Movements did not produce a step change in signal level but a prolonged and complicated transient. The initial movement signal was therefore detected and the outputs for the load cells sampled at 3 s intervals and averaged over 30 s until a stable value was obtained. The magnitude of the change in signal, and the time of the event, were both stored, allowing the characterisation of the move magnitude and the time of the event.

Direct Observation

Observation of the sleeping subject is the most direct way of obtaining movement data. Time-lapse cine-photography is a more convenient method of observation, and 6 frames per minute is a commonly used frequency (Southwell *et al.*, 1972). The technique may, however, require the use of levels of light intensity which can be expected to have a disturbing effect on sleep. This problem may be overcome by using infrared light sources either with a television and video recorder (Muzet *et al.*, 1972), or with a still camera (Bardsley *et al.*, 1976).

Time-lapse systems produce very large quantities of records for subsequent analysis, most of which show the absence of movement. Bardsley *et al.* (1976) combined photographic recording with a bed-weighing system, so that the camera was triggered and a photograph taken only when a movement had been detected.

The classification of movements from the pictures of the subject's posture also presents a problem, there being no standardised procedure.

MOVEMENT PATTERNS

Variation with Time

Patients in hospital will often be in bed, and nominally asleep, during the period 22.00 to 06.00 hours. Detailed analysis of overnight mobility records suggest that during the first and last hours the patients make an abnormally large number of movements compared with the intermediate times. This effect is apparent in the specimen data presented by Hinton (1961). For representative results required it may be better to use data obtained between 23.00 and 05.00 hours.

As has been mentioned above there is also a night-by-night variation, especially in response to patient-mounted systems. There is also evidence that a change of environment, particularly admission to hospital, produces changes in movement patterns.

Characterisation

The mobility of patients in bed can be simply characterised by the number of movements made or the number weighted, albeit unintentionally, by move magnitude as was done by Exton-Smith and Sherwin (1961). More detailed analysis can be made of the results obtained using systems which detect the time of occurrence of each movement. There is a very wide range of intermovement intervals, but the distribution is positively skewed in data obtained from normal subjects (Barbenel *et al.*, 1978), or elderly hospital patients (Figure 19.2), with the majority of the intervals being very short. The data is clearly not normally distributed but is transformed into a normal distribution if the logarithm of the time interval is used (Figure 19.3), i.e. the intermove intervals are distributed lognormally. Such distributions may, if required, be characterised by two parameters analogous to the mean and variance of the normal distribution.

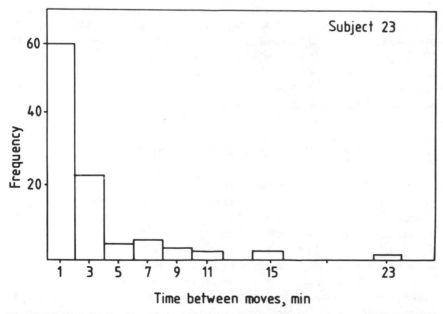

Figure 19.2 Distribution of times between movements made by elderly hospital patients. The distribution is skewed, with short intermove intervals predominating. The histogram blocks are in units of 2 min, e.g. 0–2 min

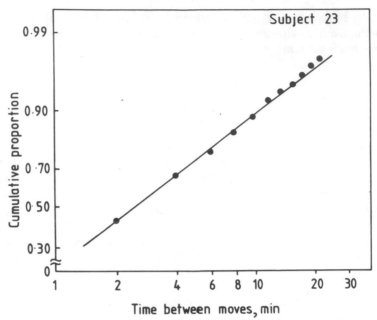

Figure 19.3   The distribution of times between movements is lognormally distributed. In the graph the abscissa is logarithmic and the ordinate the cumulant of the normal probability function

It has been suggested that only movements greater than a specific magnitude produce significant changes of interface pressure (Barbenel, 1979), and that small and large moves arise from different neurological mechanisms (Southwell *et al.*, 1972). No evidence to substantiate these differences between move sizes was found on detailed analysis of the movement data of Barbenel *et al.* (1985).

MOBILITY AND PRESSURE SORE RISK

There have been two major studies of the relationship between movements made by elderly hospital patients in bed and pressure sore risk.

Exton-Smith and Sherwin (1961) used the apparatus designed by Sherwin *et al.*, and described above, to record the number of movements made during a 7-hour period by 50 elderly patients. The bed used had, of course, a spring base and large changes in position were recorded as multiple movements. There was a strong relationship between a reduced number of movements in bed and the incidence of pressure sores. Nine of the 10 patients who made 20 or fewer movements in the recording period developed a sore. No sores occurred in any of the 28 patients who made more than 54 movements in the 7-hour monitoring period.

Despite these clear-cut conclusions, and the possibility of using the number of overnight movements to detect patients at high risk of developing sores, this work has been neither repeated nor substantiated.

Barbenel and colleagues (Barbenel *et al.*, 1985, 1986) investigated the mobility of elderly hospital patients on solid-based King's Fund beds in order to develop an instrumented process for detecting the high-risk patients. The bed-weighing system was used and data obtained for 8 hours, but the analysis was restricted to the movements recorded for the 6 hours between 23.00 and 05.00 hours. Unlike in the Exton-Smith and Sherwin study none of the patients developed a sore, and they were classified as being at high or low risk of developing sores using the Norton risk assessment system (Norton *et al.*, 1962). Results were obtained from 40 patients who were monitored for a period of 233 nights.

Hospital wards and hospital beds are less than ideal for making quantitative measurements of movement size. Analysis of the effect of floor vibration and of footfalls adjacent to the bed showed that movements resulting in changes in the position of the patient's centre of mass of less than 10 mm were not reliably detected and the analysis was based on the number of movements above this threshold.

Group comparisons of unsedated patients who could be unambiguously classified by the Norton assessment as being at high or low risk of developing sores showed statistically significant differences both between the patient groups and between the results obtained on different nights (Table 19.1). In general the results obtained on the first and second nights after admission were different from each other and from subsequent nights.

Table 19.1 Group comparisons of mobility

Measurement night	*Findings for unsedated patients (significance)*
1st	High-risk patients made fewer movements than low-risk ($p < 0.001$).
2nd	No movement difference between high- and low-risk patients ($p > 0.05$).
3rd and subsequent	High-risk patients made fewer movements than low-risk ($p < 0.001$).
1st versus 2nd	Fewer movements made on second night than first ($p < 0.001$). All low-risk patients made fewer moves on second night; high-risk patients were more variable.
	Findings for sedated and unsedated patients (significance)
3rd and subsequent	Reduction of number of movements in sedated patients High-risk patients ($p < 0.02$). Low-risk patients ($p < 0.001$).

The group comparisons confirmed that there was a correlation between mobility and pressure sore risk, but the detection of individual high-risk patients was difficult. The results did not substantiate the simple classification used by Exton-Smith and Sherwin. On the first night after admission, the high-risk patients made fewer movements than the low-risk but the marked inter-patient variability made the classification of risk by movement number unreliable with numerous misclassifications.

In developing classification criteria from mobility measurements it is important to establish what properties are required of the discrimination process. It is essential that the classification be made early in order that high-risk patients can be provided with preventive care before a sore develops. In the interest of rapid classification it was decided, to use the number of movements (n_1) recorded on the first and second (n_2) nights as the basis for the classification. The misclassification of patients as false high- or low-risk is important. At first sight it might appear that misclassifying high-risk patients as low-risk would be more undesirable than the misclassification of low-risk patients. In fact the majority of patients will be in the low-risk group and their misassignment would impose an acceptably large additional nursing load.

Analysis of the results identified three useful discriminators. Patients were classified as being at high risk of developing sores if their movement records showed that they

1. made 30 or fewer movements of the first night after admission;
2. made more movements on the second night than the first night after admission ($n_1 < n_2$); or
3. satisfied the criterion $(n_1 - 44)^2 + (n_2 - 22)^2 > (16.5)^2$.

Table 19.2 Classification patient risk

Criterion	Proportion of patients classified as high-risk from mobility measurements	
	High-risk from Norton assessment	*Low-risk from Norton assessment*
Fewer than 30 moves on night 1 (n_1)	0.7	0.19
More moves on night 2 (n_2) than night 1 (n_1)	0.6	0.19
Empirical: $(n_1 - 44)^2 + (n_2 - 22)^2 > (16.5)^2$	1.0	0.38
Majority agreement between 2 or 3 of above	0.9	0.19
	True positives	False positives

The second criterion was based on the finding that low-risk patients showed a more consistent reduction in mobility on the second night than did the high-risk patients. Criterion 3 was purely empirical, identifying all the high-risk patients. The proportion of patients classified as being at high-risk from mobility measurements are shown in Table 19.2. The majority decision based on the agreement of the results of either 2 or 3 of the criteria appeared to be most reliable. All discrimination criteria were imperfect and misclassification occurred, but this would seem to be inevitable given the multifactorial nature of pressure sore initiation.

The measurements allow the detection of movement size, but the most useful classification analysis depended only on the number of relatively large movements, and this should make it possible to design simpler systems of detection.

The study confirmed previous reports that sedatives reduced the number of movements made by patients in bed (Hinton, 1962; Exton-Smith, 1967). The comparison of patients in the high-risk group suggested that the reduction was not highly significant ($p < 0.02$), but a highly significant reduction occurred in the remainder of the patients ($p < 0.001$).

REFERENCES

Bar, C. A., Lloyd, S., Pathy, M. S. and Chawla, J. C. (1983). System to monitor gross positional changes in recumbent patients. *Care, Science and Practice*, 2(4), 4–7

Barbenel, J. C. (1979). *Research, Development and Evaluation on Improved Hospital Bed Support Surfaces and Materials.* A report to the Scottish Home and Health Department, University of Strathclyde, Glasgow

Barbenel, J. C., Jordan, M. M., Nicol, S. M. and Clark, M. O. (1977). Incidence of pressure sores in the Greater Glasgow Health Board Area. *Lancet*, ii, 548–550

Barbenel, J. C., Evans, J. H. and Jordan, M. M. (1978). Tissue mechanics. *Engineering in Medicine*, 7, 5–9

Barbenel, J. C., Ferguson-Pell, M. W. and Beale, A. Q. (1985). Monitoring the mobility of patients in bed. *Med. and Biol. Eng. and Comput.*, 23, 466–468

Barbenel, J. C., Ferguson-Pell, M. W. and Kennedy, R. (1986). Mobility of elderly patients in bed. *J. Am. Geriatr. Soc.*, 34, 633–636

Bardsley, G. I., Bell, F., and Barbenel, J. C. (1976). A technique for monitoring body movements during sleep. In Kenedi, R. M., Cowden, J. M. and Scales, J. T. (eds), *Bed Sore Biomechanics*, Macmillan Press, London and Basingstoke, pp. 225–233

Brocklehurst, J. C., Skorecki, J. and Lewis, D. (1974). Restlessness in sleep. *Eng. in Med.*, 3 (3), 10–16

Cox, G. H. and Marley, E. (1959). The estimation of motility during rest or sleep. *J. Neurol. Neurosurg. Psychiat.*, 22, 57–60

Crisp, A. H., Stonehill, E. and Eversden, I. D. (1970). The design of a mobility bed including its calibration for the subject's weight. *Med. and Biol. Engng.*, 8, 455–463

Daniel, R. K., Priest, D. L. and Wheatley, D. C. (1981). Etiological factors in pressures sores. *Arch. Phys. Med. Rehabil.*, **62**, 492–497

Exton-Smith, A. N. (1967). Use and abuse of hypnotics. *Geront. Clin.*, **9**, 264–269

Exton-Smith, A. N. and Sherwin, R. W. (1961). The prevention of pressure sores: significance of spontaneous bodily movements. *Lancet*, **ii**, 1124–1125

Feguson-Pell, M. W., Bell, F. and Evans, J. H. (1976). Interface pressure sensors. In Kenedi, R. M., Cowden, J. M. and Scales, J. T. (eds), *Bedsore Biomechanics*, Macmillan Press, London and Basingstoke, pp. 189–197

Hinton, J. M. (1961). The action of amylobarbitone sodium, butobarbitone, and quinalbarbitotone sodium upon insomnia and nocturnal restlessness, compared in psychiatric patients. *Br. J. Pharmacol.*, **16**, 82–89

Hinton, J. M. (1962). Sleep: sleep motility in depressive illness. *Proc. R. Soc. Med.*, **55**, 907–910

Jordan, M. M. and Barbenel, J. C. (1983). Pressure sore prevalance. In Barbenel, J. C., Forbes, C. D. and Lowe, G. D. O. (eds), *Pressure Sores*, Macmillan Press, London and Basingstoke, pp. 59–66

Kleitman, N. (1932). New methods for studying mobility during sleep. *Proc. Soc. Exptl. Biol. Med.*, **29**, 389–391

Korn, V., Franetzki, M. and Gottschaldt, M. (1974). Ein Verfahren zur Erfassung der patientenmotorik. *Biomedizinische Technik*, **19**, 14–19

Kresse, H. and Rettenmaier, G. (1973). Die Moderne Methodik der Sclaftiefen-messung, *Biomedizinische Technik*, **18**, 55–57

Lowthian, P. (1987). The practical assessment of pressure sore risk, *Care Science and Practice*, **5** (4), 3–7

Muzet, A. Becht, J., Jacquot, P. and Koenig, P. (1972). A technique for recording human body posture during sleep. *Pschophysiol.*, **9**, 660–662

Noble, P. C. (1981). *The Prevention of Pressure Sores in Persons with Spinal Cord Injuries*, World Rehabilitation Fund, New York

Norton, D., McLaren, R. and Exton-Smith, A. N. (1962). *An Investigation of Geriatric Nursing Problems in Hospital*, National Corporation for Care of Old People, London

Reswick, J. B. and Rogers, J. E. (1976). Experience at Rancho Los Amigos Hospital with devices and techniques to prevent pressure sores. In Kenedi, R. M., Cowden, J. M. and Scales, J. T. (eds), *Bedsore Biomechanics*, Macmillan Press, London and Basingstoke, pp. 301–310

Sherwin, R. W., Exton-Smith, A. N. and Haines, J. D. (1961). Apparatus for recording spontaneous bodily movements, *Lancet*, **ii**, 1126–1127

Southwell, P. R., Evans, C. R. and Hunt, J. N. (1972). Effect of a hot milk drink on movements during sleep. *Br. Med. J.*, **2**, 429–431

Tamura, T., Togawa, T. and Murata, M. (1988). A bed temperature monitoring system for assessing body movement during sleep. *Clin. Phys. Physiol. Meas.*, **9**, 139–145

Wheatley, D. C. (1982). *Assessment of Movement in the Elderly During Sleep with Reference to Pressure Sore Prevention*. Ph.D. Thesis, University of Strathclyde, Glasgow, UK

Wheatley, D. C., Berme, N. and Ferguson-Pell, M. W. (1982). A low profile load transducer for monitoring movement during sleep. *Experimental Mechanics*, **20**, 19–21

20

Remote Monitoring of Wheelchair Sitting Behaviour

*Martin W. Ferguson-Pell, Debra E. Hurwitz, Thomas G. Burn
and R. Masiello*

INTRODUCTION

Information about wheelchair sitting behaviour can be of great significance to the clinician wishing to maximise independence and functionality. It is ironical, however, that clinical evaluation is often undertaken in the clinic, with at best some observation while the patient 'takes a spin' down the corridor. It would seem more desirable to assimilate information while the patient is using the chair in the field under normal operational circumstances. Closer consideration of this problem presents some major engineering challenges. Not least is the identification and definition of measurable parameters that are representative of the observations made by the experienced clinician.

In this study a monitoring system is described that has been designed to measure, in the field, factors that may place a wheelchair user at risk of developing pressure sores. Pressure sores affect between 5 and 10 per cent of spinal-cord-injured wheelchair users each year (Ferguson-Pell *et al.*, 1982). The ulceration of soft tissues that is associated with pressure sore formation usually occurs over a bony area that supports the body weight of the patient. In the sitting position the bony areas at risk include the ischial tuberosities, the sacrum and the posterior aspect of the greater trochanters. Pressure sores are thought to develop following periods of prolonged ischaemia to the soft tissues when bearing body weight, for example while sitting. The wheelchair user at risk is normally trained to relieve pressure to these tissues periodically, normally by supporting body weight on the arms (push-up) or by rocking sideways. The recommended frequency and duration of pressure relief activities appears to have evolved from collective clinical experience and is normally quoted as a complete relief every 10 minutes for 10 seconds. There appears to be little physiological evidence to support these figures and it seems likely that individuals have different needs for ischaemia relief in order to remain at low risk for developing pressure sores. This is discussed further in Chapter 15. There is also little or no evidence that once discharged from hospital spinal-cord-injured persons actually follow the pressure relief prescription given to them; the

261

connection between actual performance and the recommended frequency and duration of pressure relief is therefore unknown.

It is the authors' thesis that careful evaluation of actual pressure relief performance, and other parameters describing sitting behaviour, would assist in developing an understanding of the real conditions that are tolerated without breakdown. In a more extensive study, producing a large database of sitting behaviour, it should also be possible to correlate actual performance of pressure relief activity with pressure sore incidence. The importance of pressure relief activity could be determined, and recommended frequencies for pressure relief established on the basis of objective data.

Parameters of interest include the following:

1. average frequency of pressure reliefs;
2. average duration of pressure reliefs;
3. variation in (1) and (2) with time of day and day of week;
4. evidence for asymmetry in pressure relief behaviour favouring relief to one side if performing lateral leans;
5. evidence for asymmetry in tissue loading resulting from habitual sitting behaviour.

Previous studies provide us with some insight into sitting performance in the hospital environment. Fisher and Patterson (1983) developed a system for monitoring pressure beneath the ischial tuberosities, recording data continuously for up to 24 hours using a small portable tape recorder. The pressure transducers were attached directly to the patient's skin, thereby limiting the study to an environment in which the transducers and recorder could be continuously maintained. The data in this study confirmed, however, that most subjects sat for well in excess of the prescribed interval before performing pressure reliefs. In fact, many sat for well in excess of 1 hour between relief events. This study did provide some evidence for asymmetric sitting behaviour that was not detected during the routine clinical evaluation of the patient.

Merbitz and co-workers (1983, 1985) have developed a computer-based Timer Logger Communicator (TLC) employing switches placed in the wheelchair cushion. In this study serial monitoring sessions allowed a composite picture of sitting behaviour to be developed for up to 28 days in a hospital setting. The instrumentation placed several constraints on the study. The sensors limit the variety of cushion types that can be used to those that allow the switch to be inserted into the cushion material. Air-filled and other fluid-filled cushions are not ideally suited to the TLC monitoring system. The hard-wire connection between the sensors and the monitoring electronics require some user intervention in the form of either disconnection of the electronics pack from the sensors, or else removal of the sensors from the cushion. This is undesirable, as a long-term monitoring session should not rely on technical intervention from the subject. There is likely to be a statistical link between the patient's reliability in supporting the monitor technically and compliance in performing pressure reliefs. Merbitz *et al.* (1985) do however confirm that many of their patients experience prolonged periods of ischaemia without immediate evidence of tissue breakdown. Although the TLC does extend the work of Patterson and Fisher in providing a more readily applied clinical tool, this is accomplished at the cost of collecting samples of habitual sitting symmetry.

In neither of the above studies does the instrumentation permit free-ranging data acquisition without technical support for more than 24 hours. The authors of this study have therefore established that a suitable device should:

1. Be capable of operating for longer than 30 days without the need for technical intervention either to recharge the power supply or to transfer data to free-up computer memory.
2. Require no user intervention throughout the monitoring period.
3. Allow the patient's own wheelchair and cushion system to be used without major disassembly or modification.
4. Remain accurate throughout the normal range of environmental changes for an active wheelchair user, namely room temperature range from 0 °C to 40 °C and relative humidity up to 100 per cent.
5. Be sufficiently robust to withstand minor mechanical impacts during wheelchair propulsion over rough terrain or during transportation, for example by baggage handlers.
6. Be capable of measuring the parameters of interest listed above.

DESIGN CONSIDERATIONS

Our concept for a monitoring device to meet the above specifications was to develop a portable wheelchair seat force plate. The signal conditioning and data acquisition system would be attached to the underside of the force plate, the whole system supported on hooks resting on the frame of the wheelchair. The only modification to the wheelchair would be the replacement of the canvas sling seat by the force plate for the duration of the study. Drop seats, whereby a plywood platform is suspended on hooks, are widely used by clinicians wishing to control the sitting height of their patient when using extra-thick cushions in association with work surfaces having normal leg clearance.

This approach provides an opportunity for a portable, robust design that can accommodate all types of wheelchair cushions and can be fitted, with minor adjustments, to most commercially produced wheelchairs. By monitoring not only the vertical force component on the plate but also the centre of pressure of the sitting subject it is possible to detect with a high degree of accuracy both push-up and lateral-lean types of pressure relief. Furthermore by periodically sampling sitting position it is possible to obtain a measure for habitual asymmetric sitting. The individual with a tendency to sit off-centre on the seat, but who loads each buttock equally, can be differentiated from the individual who tends to lean to one side, by measuring the skewness of the sampled centre of pressure distribution about its mean. The off-centre sitter will have a low level of skewness and a mean centre of pressure position that does not correspond to the axis of symmetry of the seat. The asymmetric sitter will generate a higher level of skewness about an arbitary mean position on the seat.

Although conceptually simple, this approach presents some significant technical challenges. In order that the system functions for at least 30 days the power consumption of both the force-plate signal conditioning and the data acquisition system must be very low. Since a significant event is unpredictable and 1 second or longer in duration (Merbitz *et al.*, 1983, 1985) the system must be capable of virtually continuous 'listening' for events while also being able to sample the position of the subject's centre of pressure in order to develop the frequency distribution needed to test for skewness. Although a piezoelectric force plate transducer system offers the advantages of negligible power consumption and would be capable of measuring events associated with a change in sitting status (push-up, side lean) it would not accurately reflect the position of the centre of pressure of the subject during quasi-static phases of sitting. We therefore felt constrained to use traditional strain-gauged force sensors placed at each corner of the plate, each configured as a Wheatstone bridge.

The net power consumption of this configuration can be readily limited by using short-pulse-width energization, sampling at a frequency of 2 Hz in order to capture significant events. Unfortunately the instrumentation amplifiers necessary to amplify the small bridge voltages involved use significant power to operate. In this study we elected to use a low-power bipolar instrumentation amplifier but to operate it with a power supply that was pulsed in synchronization with the bridge energisation. We discovered that although a very unconventional approach, the amplifier tolerated a square-wave pulse as short as 5 ms without distortion or significant loss of output stability.

None of the microprocessors that we reviewed were capable of operating continuously in the tens of microamperes range needed to limit our 1-month power consumption to the 3 A h available in D-cell-sized high-energy-capacity batteries. We therefore decided that the data acquisition circuitry should remain off until a significant event occurs or it is time for another sample to be taken of the subject's sitting position. This was accomplished by allowing event detection circuitry to control the power supply to the computer. When a significant event occurs the computer's power supply is turned on by transistors and the computer rapidly operates software stored on an EPROM. Data from the force transducers is sampled by the computer's A–D converter and processed to classify the event. Significant events are encoded, time-stamped and stored in the 64K, battery-backed-up CMOS RAM of the computer circuit.

In order for the analogue circuitry to determine that an event is of sufficient magnitude and duration to justify 'waking up' the computer, preprocessing is performed. This is accomplished by using a series of summer circuits and an analogue divider that satisfy the following equations:

$$X = K_1(F_1 + F_2)/(F_1 + F_2 + F_3 + F_4),$$
$$Y = K_2(F_2 + F_3)/(F_1 + F_2 + F_3 + F_4),$$
$$W = (F_1 + F_2 + F_3 + F_4),$$

where K_1 and K_2 are constants defined by the geometry of the force plate and W is the weight of the subject supported by the seat. F_1–F_4 are the forces measured by each of the force transducers on the force plate.

Level detectors are used to define thresholds (T) for the voltages corresponding to X, Y and W to define right and left pressure relief leans ($T_{right} > X > T_{left}$); forward leans ($Y > T_{forward}$) or push-up ($W < T_{push-up}$). Counters are used to determine that an event is longer than 1 second before activating the computer.

Although the level detectors are used to 'wake up' the computer, the system does not rely on them to classify events accurately. For each subject, at the beginning of the monitoring period a calibration procedure is followed while interface pressure is monitored using a simple pneumatic transducer (Talley Medical, Borehamwood) under the ischial tuberosities. The subject is asked to follow his normal sequence of push-ups and lateral leans while being monitored by the computer. Loci for the centre of pressure values are determined which define each of the pressure relief events and are stored in RAM. When an event occurs the computer compares the incoming force transducer values (F_{1-4}) with the thresholds. If a valid pressure relief event for the subject being monitored is detected then it is time-stamped and recorded, otherwise it is ignored and the computer switches off.

The design of the force plate presented many difficulties. It was required to be lightweight yet capable of measuring accurately for up to a month without significant drift or errors associated with temperature or humidity changes. It was required to attach safely to the frame of the wheelchair without mechanical modification yet be insensitive to the inherent flexing of the wheelchair. A four-transducer design was selected to solve the above equations without adjustment for the subject's weight. A simple, doubly-supported beam design was selected (Figure 20.1) for ease of fabrication, high sensitivity to vertical-force components and low lateral-force

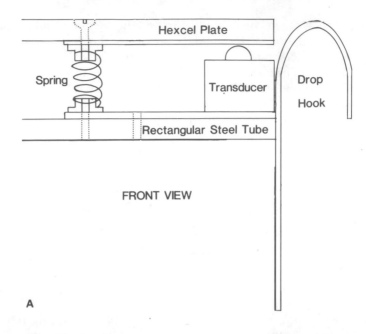

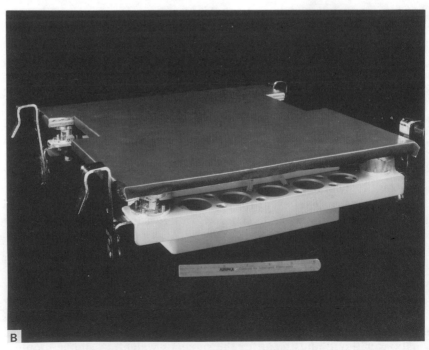

Figure 20.1 (A) Diagrammatic representation of the force plate. (B) Illustration of PRAM system

sensitivity. The transducers are mechanically decoupled from the supporting structure of the force plate by a silicon adhesive, ensuring that the wheelchair frame flexion has a negligible effect on the transducer output. A spring and connecting-rod system is used to maintain the relative location of the top plate and the transducer support tube/hook assembly. The top plate is fabricated from Hexcel, a honeycomb aluminium material affording light weight and high rigidity, and transmits loading to the force transducer through a plastic sphere to decouple in-plane forces. Adjustment to the overall width of the system is provided by attaching the support hooks to rectangular rods which pass through a rectangular tube fitted with locking bolts. The system allows for a range of wheelchair widths from 350 to 500 mm, using a set of three easily interchanged Hexcel plates. The electronics package is supported underneath the top plate and attached with Velcro to facilitate easy removal when replacing the top plate to accommodate different widths of wheelchair.

PERFORMANCE OF MONITORING SYSTEM

The pressure relief and asymmetry monitor (PRAM) has been thoroughly evaluated in order to meet the original specifications.

Temperature Stability

The PRAM monitoring system was placed in an environmental chamber and subjected to an increase in temperature from 0 to 38 °C while operating in continuous-output mode, each output channel being monitored by a strip chart recorder. Figure 20.2(A) indicates the variation in the X- and Y-coordinates of the centre of pressure as the environmental temperature was increased. Figure 20.2(B) indicates the equivalent change in output, expressed in calibrated force units (N), with change in temperature.

Linearity

The system was loaded with known weights applied at the centre of the plate. Figure 20.3 indicates the linearity of the load versus output on the W-channel. A specified weight was then placed at points 50 mm apart along the axes of symmetry of the plate to determine its linearity with position of loading. The results plotting position versus the output on the X- and Y-channels is presented in Figure 20.4.

A further test was performed to determine the sensitivity of the system to position for a fixed weight. Ideally the plate should record the same

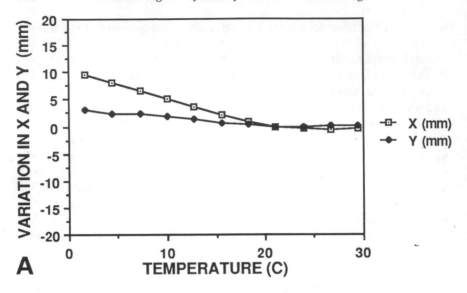

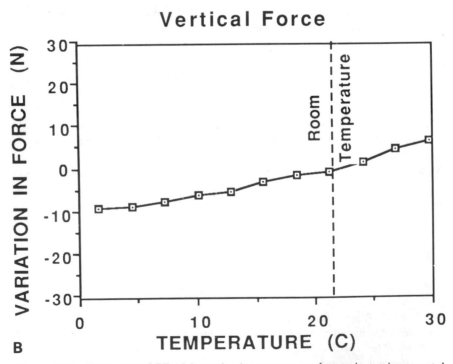

Figure 20.2   Response of PRAM monitoring system to change in environmental temperature. (A) Variation in output representing *X*- and *Y*-coordinates of centre of pressure. (B) Variation in output for constant applied weight (*F*)

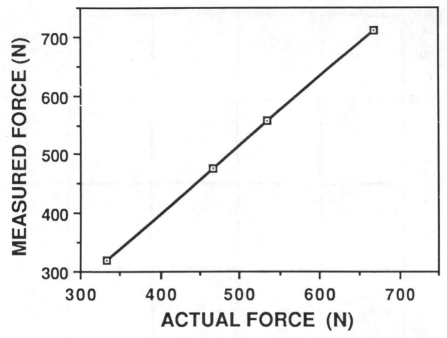

Figure 20.3 Calibration of weight channel output with applied loads at centre of force plate

value of *W* irrespective of its location on the plate. Figure 20.5 indicates the variation expressed in calibrated force units (N) for a fixed applied weight of 454 N. However, within acceptable limits, this range of output variations, i.e. 436–463 N, can be attributable to cross-talk between transducers resulting from flexion in the wheelchair and the top plate.

Weight of System

The total weight of the PRAM system is 4.8 kg. This is composed of the force plate weighing 2.8 kg, and the 2.0 kg electronics package.

Power Consumption

The PRAM is powered by two sets of D-cell-sized lithium batteries, one set for the analogue and the other for the computer circuitry. Each of these circuits is provided with a 6 V regulated supply able to deliver 3 A h. For normal estimated usage the system provides well in excess of the 1-month power capability needed to meet the specifications.

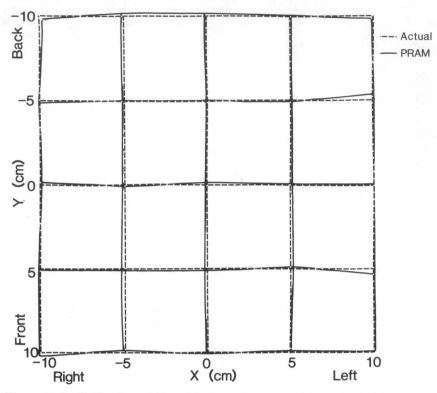

Figure 20.4   Calibration of *X*- and *Y*-channel outputs with applied load moved in
50 mm increments

Analogue circuit continuously pulsed operation requires 60 mA for each 5
ms pulse at 1 Hz (equivalent to 300 μA continuous non-pulsed), yielding
over 400 days capacity.

Computer circuit requires 60 mA when activated. Assume 1 event every 10
minutes +1 sample every 5 minutes (18 events/h) for 14 h per day. Each
event is sampled for 15 s. Power consumed per day = 63 mA h. Therefore computer circuit has 47 days capacity.

RAM Memory Capacity

Each event requires 8 bytes for classification and time stamping. At a rate
of 250 events/samples per day (see power consumption calculation above),
the system would fill the 60K data storage space in the RAM in 30 days. It
is therefore possible that very active subjects will fill the RAM within the
30 day deadline. The data from Merbitz *et al.* (1983, 1985) and Fisher and

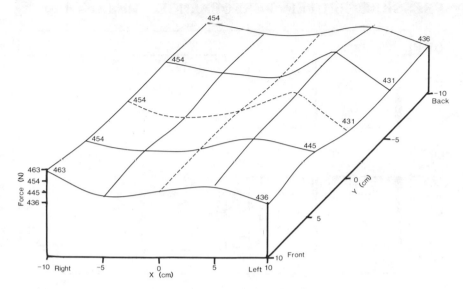

Figure 20.5 Response of force plate weight channel to a single load applied at different points on the surface of the plate

Patterson (1983) however suggest a typical activity level that is much lower than the prescribed 'ideal' used above.

Data Presentation

In order to display the data collected by PRAM's Z-80 CMOS microprocessor system, software has been developed by the authors to display the data for clinical interpretation. Data stored in PRAM's RAM is transferred to a personal computer (IBM PC or compatible) at the end of a monitoring session using two communication software packages, Kermit and Xmodem. Error checking is performed by Xmodem to ensure accuracy during the transfer.

A graphical display of the data using software developed by the authors in the C programming language allows the type duration and frequency of pressure relief to be readily visualised. A horizontal scrolling feature allows the user to trace activity along the time continuum. Figure 20.6 provides a typical example of data collected using PRAM for a 4-hour period.

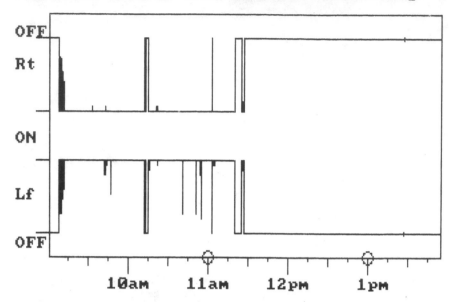

Figure 20.6　Processed data from a short PRAM monitoring session as presented to the investigator on the personal computer display. Each event is recorded as a vertical line, the length of which is proportional to the duration of the event. The interval between events can be determined from the horizontal axis. If both the right and left traces record the event it is a push-up. If a lateral lean is performed, only a single vertical line is displayed, indicating to which side the subject leaned

DISCUSSION

A monitoring system is described which resolves many of the technical difficulties experienced to date in monitoring aspects of wheelchair sitting performance related to the problem of pressure sores. The activities associated with pressure activities are sufficiently infrequent to permit long-term monitoring using a system with 64K memory. The power consumption of the system is well within the required tolerances for this application. Taking a broader view of wheelchair performance monitoring, it is clear that a system capable of capturing more rapidly occurring events would encounter major problems balancing limited power capacity and memory requirements. In such circumstances it would seem desirable to undertake studies with technical staff in the field using telemetry or umbilical systems to monitor transient events.

The next phase in the application of the PRAM system will be its implementation in full clinical trials. Studies are planned to investigate changes in pressure relief performance associated with two 'interventions'.

In the first, patients will be monitored prior to discharge during rehabilitation for spinal-cord injury and then again in the field once they have left hospital. We hope to determine how much change in compliance with their pressure relief regimen can be attributed to the distractions of the home and workplace. In the second we will evaluate the effect that an educational programme teaching pressure sore prevention techniques has on actual pressure relief activity for both hospital and community-based spinal-cord-injured persons.

ACKNOWLEDGEMENTS

Helen Hayes Hospital is operated by the New York State Department of Health.

REFERENCES

Ferguson-Pell, M. W., Wilkie, I. C., Reswick, J. B. and Barbenel, J. C. (1982). Pressure sore prevention for the wheelchair-bound spinal cord injured patient. *Paraplegia*, **18**, 42–51
Fisher, S. V. and Patterson, P. (1983). Long term pressure recordings under the ischial tuberosities of tetraplegics. *Paraplegia*, **21**, 99–106
Merbitz, C. T., King, R. B. and Bleiberg, J. (1983). Continuous direct recording of wheelchair pressure relief behavior. *Arch. Phys. Med. Rehabil.*, **64** (Abstr.), 490–491
Merbitz, C. T., King, R. M., Bleiberg, J. and Grip, J. (1985). Wheelchair push-ups: measuring pressure relief frequency. *Arch. Phys. Med. Rehabil.*, **66**, 433–438

Index